I0704811

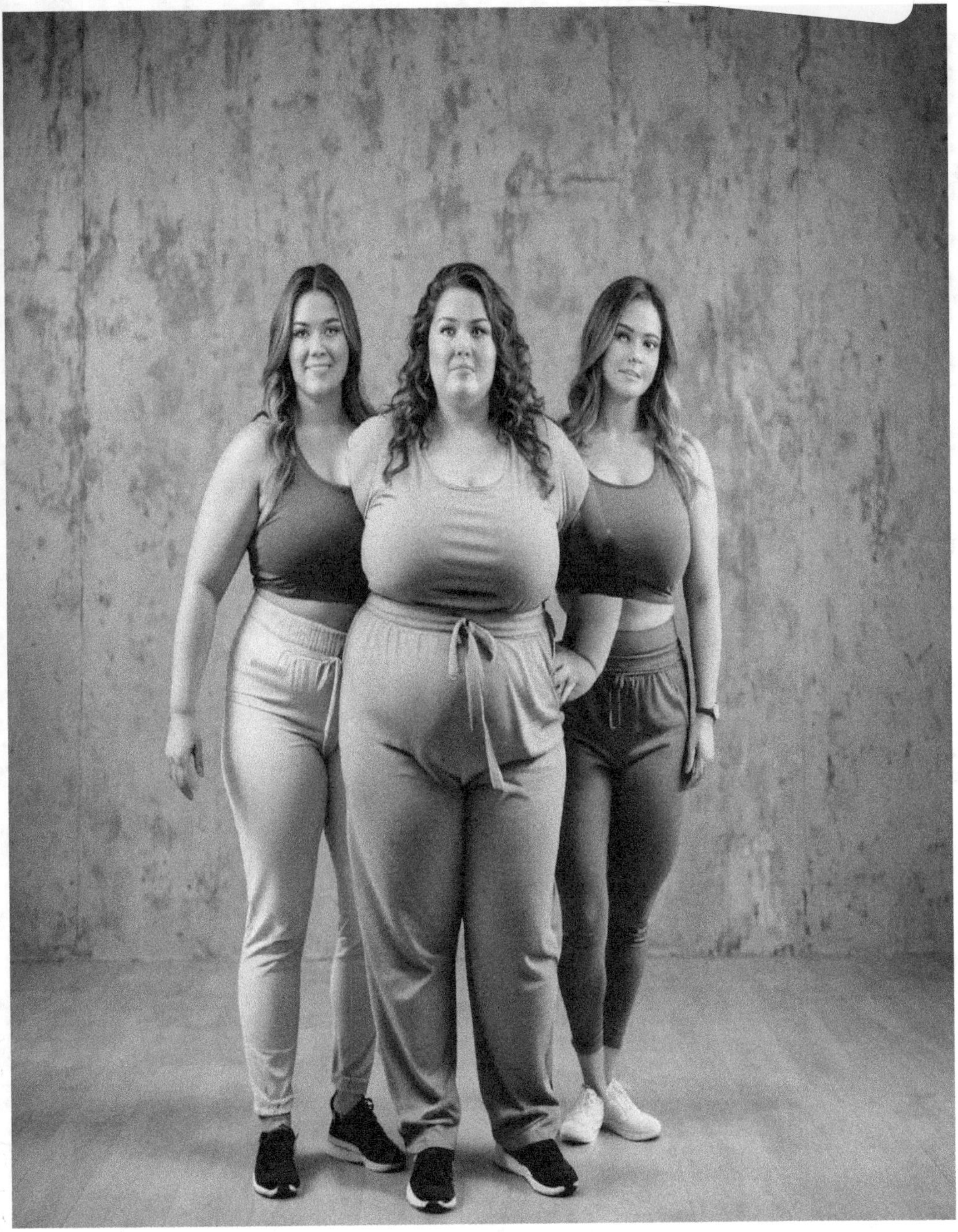

Table of Contents

Shedding the Myths
Unveiling the Science of Weight Loss

by

David Holman

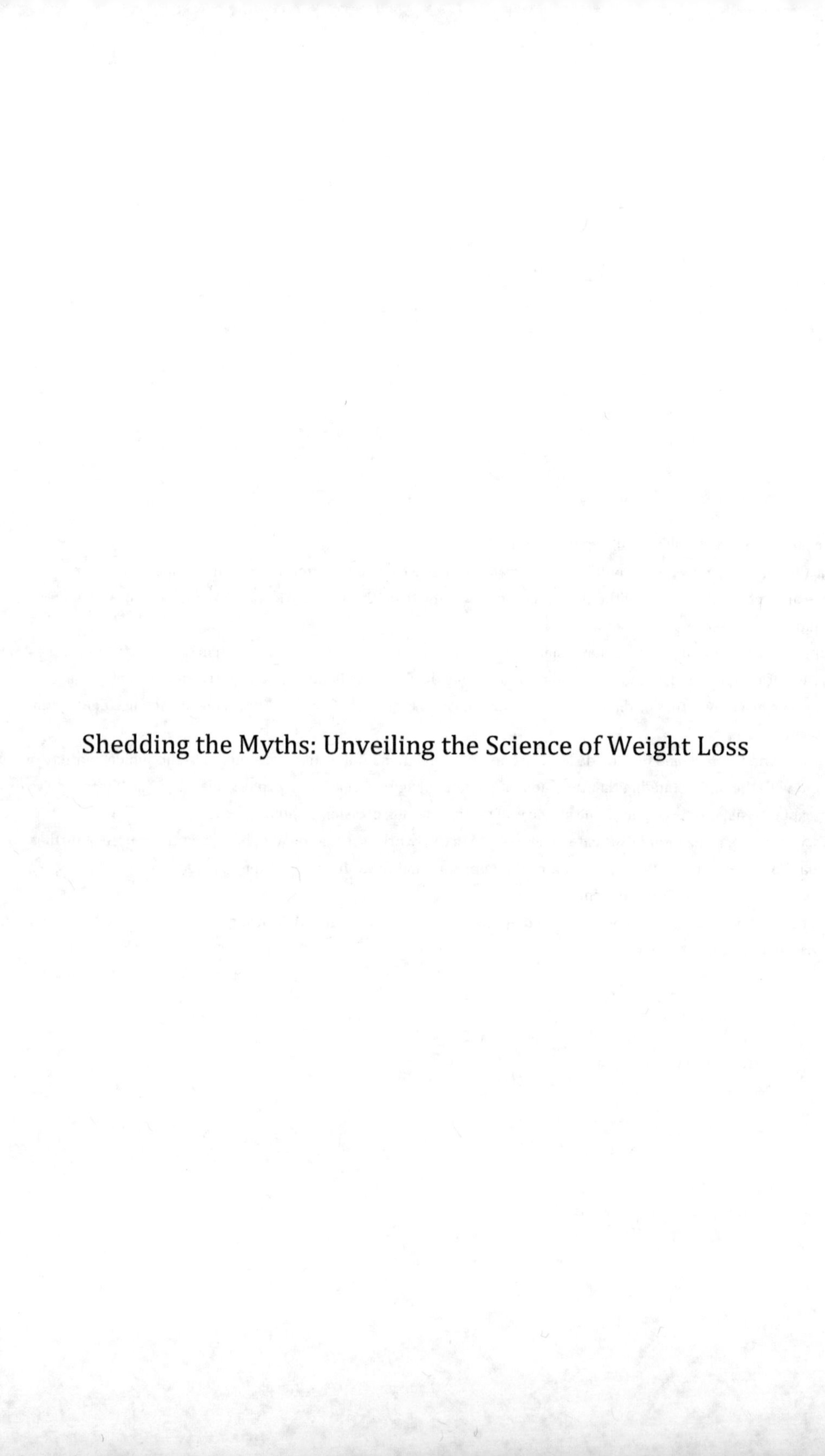

Shedding the Myths: Unveiling the Science of Weight Loss

Contents

Introduction

In a world fitfully obsessed with dietary trends and fitness regimes, weight loss remains a deeply personal and often challenging journey. It's an endeavor not just of the body but also of the mind and spirit. The notion that achieving and maintaining a healthy weight could be simplified to a formula of "eat less, move more" has long been dismantled by the complexities of human biology, emotions, and lifestyle. So, why a book on weight loss amidst the cacophony of quick fixes? Because this is not about losing weight for a season but about nurturing a way of living that enriches your life.

At the core of this journey is the understanding of oneself, one's habits, and one's environment. The goal here isn't to provide you with another set of rigid rules or a magical diet that promises instant results. Instead, we aim to empower you with knowledge and tools that honor your unique biological makeup and lifestyle. The chapters ahead explore a holistic approach to weight loss that integrates proven scientific insights, critical lifestyle changes, and mindful practices that foster a healthier relationship with food, exercise, and oneself.

Weight loss, as we see it, is not merely about shedding pounds. It's about shedding the burdens of misinformation, unrealistic expectations, and the unrelenting pressure of societal norms. This book respects you as an individual with complex needs and strives to meet those needs by providing information that's both grounded in science and compassionate in understanding the human experience. It's about creating a sustainable lifestyle that supports your physical and mental well-being well beyond the point where the scales tip in your favor.

We begin by touching on the intricacies of metabolism and the often misunderstood role genetics play. Here, you'll learn why some people can eat more without gaining weight and why that doesn't mean all efforts are futile if you're not in that group. Science has provided us with fascinating insights into how our bodies work, but what's more critical is how we apply these insights in real life. Throughout the book, you'll find actionable strategies that help you make informed decisions rather than reactive ones.

Nutrition is another cornerstone of this journey. You'll be introduced to the essential roles macronutrients play and how a balanced approach can be the key to unlocking both health and satisfaction. It's not about deprivation; it's about making choices that serve both your health goals and your palate. You'll discover how meal timing can influence weight management and realize that every choice and habit creates ripples in your body's nutritional landscape.

Exercise also plays its part but not as a tool of punishment or a trade-off for food indulgences. The chapters dedicated to physical activity will illustrate how the right kind of exercise not only aids in weight loss but also becomes a joyful and integral part of your daily routine. By understanding the role of cardio and strength training, you can create an empowering exercise regimen that suits your aspirations and physical capabilities.

Beyond the physical components, this book delves into the psychological aspects of eating, an area often overlooked in quick-fix solutions. Emotional eating, stress, and the lack of mindfulness can derail the best of intentions. These insights will equip you with the ability to identify triggers, navigate cravings, and cultivate a deeper awareness of why and how you eat, which is as important as what you eat.

Moreover, sleep and stress are integral to weight management, often influencing hormones and food choices significantly. The importance of quality sleep and effective stress management techniques will be highlighted as simple yet crucial components of your weight loss toolkit.

This journey is never a solitary one. The importance of building a strong support system cannot be overstated. Whether it's family, friends, or professionals, having a network to guide, encourage, and sometimes challenge you is invaluable. The following chapters will present ways to cultivate these crucial connections that enhance your journey toward a healthier you.

Progress is not always linear, and setbacks are inevitable. However, determining how to effectively measure and interpret your progress can help sustain motivation. By learning to track your journey accurately and set realistic goals, you'll find a concrete path towards sustaining the changes you make. This becomes essential when facing plateaus or times when progress seems elusive.

Finally, we arrive at the steps necessary to cement these changes so they're not fleeting, but permanent elements of your life. It's about crafting a lifestyle, not just undergoing an experience. We offer guidance on integrating changes seamlessly and adapting them to fit the uniqueness of your life.

As you read the stories of transformation shared within these pages, remember that each story started with an individual much like you, who made a decision to embark on a transformative journey. Their success can serve as inspiration, proving that with the right tools and mindset, sustainable weight loss is achievable for anyone willing to commit to understanding and improving themselves.

In this book, you'll find the means to create a healthier, happier, and more vibrant version of yourself. Your journey towards effective and sustainable weight loss begins here, grounded in respect for science and for the strength you possess.

Chapter 1: Understanding Weight Loss

To genuinely embrace a journey of weight loss, one must begin with understanding the complex tapestry that underpins it. Weight loss is much more than a straightforward equation of eating less and moving more. It's a multifaceted process influenced by our biology, environment, and the decisions we make. By unraveling these layers, we empower ourselves to make informed choices that lead to sustainable change.

First, let's consider the science behind why we lose or gain weight. At its core, weight management involves a delicate balance between calories consumed and calories burned. This balance, however, is significantly affected by our individual metabolic rates. Metabolism is the body's engine, converting food into energy. It involves a series of chemical reactions that are influenced by genes, lifestyle, and even the food we eat. Understanding how our body uses energy and the various factors that can affect this process is crucial to managing our weight effectively.

Beneath the surface of metabolism, genetics plays an intriguing role in weight management. Many of us have heard someone say, "It's in my genes" when referring to their body shape or size. While genetics indeed have a say in the body's predisposition to store or burn fat, they are not the sole dictators of our destiny. Separating genetic influence from lifestyle choices requires introspection and honesty about our daily habits and routines. Acknowledging this dance between nature and nurture can be empowering, as it highlights areas where we can exert control and make positive changes.

Another integral aspect is understanding how psychological and social factors intertwine with physiological processes. Stress, emotions, and social influences are powerful forces that impact our eating behaviors and weight. Whether it's the comfort of food in times of stress or the communal aspect of sharing meals, these influences can steer us off course if not recognized and managed. By cultivating awareness and implementing mindful practices, we become architects of our own eating habits, laying a foundation that supports both our mental and physical well-being.

Finally, it's important to dispel the myth that rapid weight loss solutions are sustainable in the long run. Quick fixes are appealing, with promises of swift results, but these often come at the expense of long-term health. Sustainable weight loss involves gradual, consistent changes that integrate seamlessly into daily life. It's about building a lifestyle that emphasizes balance, nourishment, and enjoyment, not deprivation. By moving away from fads and embracing a more holistic approach, we pave the path for lasting change.

As we embark on this exploration of weight loss, remember that the journey is uniquely yours. It's grounded in knowledge, bolstered by resilience, and enriched by the wisdom of understanding oneself. By committing to this process, you're not just working towards weight loss; you're learning to embrace a healthier and more harmonious life.

Exploring the Science Behind Metabolism

When we talk about weight loss, metabolism often takes center stage. It seems almost mystical in how it affects our bodies, yet at its core, metabolism is a simple concept: it's how your body converts food into energy. But as straightforward as that sounds, the science of metabolism is both intricate and fascinating. By understanding it, you get one step closer to achieving lasting weight loss.

Metabolism is made up of two key processes: anabolism and catabolism. Anabolism is all about building and storing. It's the process responsible for growth, building cells, and storing energy for later use. On the other hand, catabolism is the burning of energy. This is where those stored resources are broken down to power your movements, thoughts, and all those involuntary actions that keep you alive. These processes are constantly balancing each other to maintain healthy functioning.

What's key to grasping metabolism's role in weight loss is your basal metabolic rate (BMR). BMR is the number of calories your body needs to maintain basic physiological functions like breathing, circulation, and cell production while at rest. Essentially, it's the energy cost of living. While you might think screaming cardio sessions are what melt pounds away, up to 70% of the calories you burn each day comes from BMR.

So, what influences your BMR? A few factors include age, sex, and muscle mass. As you age, muscle mass tends to decrease, which can slow down your metabolic rate. This conveys the larger picture of why exercise, especially strength training, is crucial—it helps maintain and even boost your metabolism by preserving muscle mass. Furthermore, genetics do play a role, and while you can't change your DNA, you can modify your lifestyle to work with it rather than against it.

It's also important to understand the term "metabolic rate" with nuance. Many people often conflate a "fast" metabolism with an inability to gain weight and a "slow" metabolism with weight challenges. But everyone has their unique set point. Rather than try to rev your metabolism to mythical speeds, focus on strategies that naturally align your metabolic rate with your health goals. This might mean adjusting your caloric intake or incorporating more physical activity into your daily routine.

Understanding metabolism helps demystify the mechanics behind weight loss. It's not about turning to extreme measures, but about nurturing and optimizing your body's natural processes. Knowledge is empowering—it allows you to move away from quick fixes and fads, embracing a long-term approach to weight loss that's sustainable and effective. The intricate dance of metabolism is not our foe. Instead, it's a system to partner with, guiding us towards a healthier, more balanced lifestyle.

How Metabolic Rates Affect Weight Loss Metabolic rate serves as the unseen engine of weight management, tirelessly converting the food we eat into the energy that fuels our daily activities. When we talk about metabolism, it's easy to boil it down to a simple equation of calories in versus calories out. However, the reality is far more intricate. By diving into the science behind it, we unlock a wealth of knowledge that redefines how we approach weight loss, making it less about restriction and more about understanding. Metabolism isn't uniform for everyone; it's a unique tapestry woven from your biology, lifestyle, and nutrition. At its core, metabolic rate boils down to three main components: Basal Metabolic Rate (BMR), the thermic effect of food, and physical activity. The BMR represents the largest share of your daily energy expenditure—essentially the calories you burn at rest just to keep your body functioning. The magic of BMR is that it accounts for about 60-75% of your daily calorie burn and is influenced by factors like age, gender, muscle mass, and genetic makeup. Simply put, it's why some people can eat more without gaining weight, while others gain weight with seemingly the same diet.

One of the key insights into metabolism is understanding that muscle mass significantly impacts the BMR. Muscle tissue burns more calories at rest compared to fat tissue. This explains why strength training, which we'll dive into later, is a potent ally in weight management. Building lean muscle mass through resistance exercises boosts your body's resting energy demands, subtly shifting that delicate energy equation in your favor. While the actual number of extra calories burned per pound of muscle is modest, over time, this accumulates, offering a steady path to sustainable weight loss.

It's not just about the hardware, though; the software matters too. The thermic effect of food—how much energy your body expends digesting and metabolizing food—plays a surprisingly important role. Proteins demand more caloric energy for digestion compared to fats and carbohydrates, meaning a well-balanced diet with adequate protein intake can subtly enhance your metabolic rate. This isn't to suggest a protein-only diet, but to highlight the efficiency of balanced meals that respect your body's complexity. Coupling this with mindful eating habits can exponentially improve the way you engage with food, encouraging a more intuitive understanding of your hunger and satiety signals.

Physical activity is the most variable part of your daily energy expenditure, and its impact on metabolism can't be overstated. Regular exercise not only increases the calories burned during the activity itself but also offers a post-exercise metabolic boost, known as excess post-exercise oxygen consumption (EPOC). This is where effective planning comes into play. A well-rounded exercise routine that blends cardio with strength training optimizes this process, propelling progress and staving off the dreaded plateau. It's not about punishing routines or clocking endless hours at the gym; rather, it's about consistency and finding movements you enjoy.

Understanding the sensitivity of metabolism to diet and activity highlights the importance of recognizing it as a dynamic system. Crash diets that significantly slash caloric intake can be more harmful than helpful. They can trigger a metabolic slowdown—your body entering a conservation mode, burning fewer calories in response to perceived deprivation. This adaptive thermogenesis is why many find themselves on a frustrating weight loss plateau after an initial rapid loss, followed by the rebound effect. It's a lesson in metabolic empathy, urging us to choose grace over haste in the journey to weight loss.

Moreover, let's consider the broader context of lifestyle choices. Sleep, stress, and daily habits, while appearing peripheral, wield a substantial influence on your metabolic rate. Quality rest supports hormonal balance, ensuring leptin and ghrelin—the hormones regulating hunger and fullness—are in check. Chronic stress, on the other hand, can induce hormonal disturbances that prompt your body to cling to fat, particularly around the midsection. Hence, aligning your lifestyle to support metabolic health isn't just smart—it's necessary for long-term success.

The interplay between metabolism and weight loss underscores the narrative that weight management is not a one-size-fits-all endeavor. It's about tuning into your body's unique rhythm and responding with informed choices, patience, and persistence. The key to unlocking effortless weight management lies in fostering metabolic flexibility—the ability of your body to switch efficiently between fuels, depending on availability and demand. It's akin to teaching your body to dance effortlessly between feasting and fasting, exertion and rest.

This perspective empowers us to quiet the noise of fad diets and quick fixes, embracing instead the sustainable habit changes that honor the science of metabolism. By doing so, we're not just losing weight; we're weaving a lifestyle that supports our well-being in the long run. Through the cultivation of an understanding of your metabolic landscape, you're equipped to make choices that are grounded in science rather than desperation. Now, as you move through this journey of understanding and transformation, remember that these insights are your companion, not your master. They guide you in crafting a life of health and balance, one that recognizes the profound interplay of biology, behavior, and belief. As we integrate these insights into our daily choices, the daunting task of weight loss becomes less about battling our biology and more about partnering with it. The beauty of this journey isn't just in reaching a specific number on the scale but in fostering a harmonious relationship with our bodies, founded on knowledge, respect, and compassion. In understanding how metabolic rates affect weight loss, we embrace both the science and the art of nurturing ourselves toward the lives we deserve, rejecting the shortcuts for a meaningful, lasting change.

The Role of Genetics in Weight Management

When it comes to weight management, genetics can feel like a mystery wrapped in a puzzle. For many of us, the thought that our DNA holds sway over our waistlines is as daunting as it is fascinating. But let's break it down. Our genes certainly play a role in determining body weight, influencing elements like metabolism, fat storage, and even our hunger signals. Some folks may find it easier to maintain a healthy weight due to these genetic factors, while others might struggle with weight gain despite similar lifestyle choices. Yet, it's crucial to remember that genes aren't destiny, and understanding their influence can empower us to make informed choices about our health.

Our genetic makeup can affect how our bodies respond to various nutrients and how efficiently we burn calories. For instance, certain genes are linked to a higher propensity for storing fat, while others might predispose someone to a faster metabolism. Despite these differences, studies have shown that lifestyle factors such as diet and exercise can often mitigate the influence of genetics. This means that while you may have inherited a tendency to store fat easily, balancing caloric intake with regular physical activity can shift the scales in your favor.

But where do we draw the line between genetics and lifestyle? It's a complex interplay. Key contributors include the FTO gene, often dubbed the 'fat gene,' which has been associated with increased hunger levels and calorie intake, especially from high-fat foods. However, even those with variations in this gene can achieve weight goals by embracing consistent healthy eating patterns and exercise regimens. This speaks to the power of perseverance and the choices we make daily, which can override predisposed genetic influences.

So, how do we use this information to our advantage? Firstly, understanding that genetics is but one piece of the weight management puzzle can lift a considerable burden of blame off our shoulders. With this knowledge, we can approach weight loss with strategies tailored to our unique bodies. Personalized nutrition and exercise programs, sometimes guided by genetic testing, are becoming more accessible, making it easier to formulate a plan that aligns with both our genetic makeup and our personal goals.

Moreover, acknowledging the genetic aspects of weight doesn't have to be discouraging. Instead, it can be incredibly motivating. Realizing that while we start with a genetic blueprint, the structure we build is based entirely on the daily choices we make. When confronted with setbacks or a slower-than-expected progress, it helps to know that genetics is just one of the hurdles, and it can be managed with dedication and the right strategies.

In conclusion, while our genes play a role in weight management, they don't have the final say. By embracing this knowledge, we can move forward with an approach that's informed and optimistic. Our genes may set the stage, but we're the ones who perform the script of our weight management journey. With a balanced, adaptive approach, lasting weight loss becomes an achievable goal for anyone, regardless of genetic predispositions.

Separating Genetic Influence from Lifestyle Choices In the pursuit of understanding weight loss, one of the most intricate puzzles revolves around the influence of genetics versus lifestyle choices. It can be tempting to attribute our weight entirely to our genetic makeup or, conversely, to the choices we make each day. However, the reality lies somewhere in between, where both strands play significant and often intertwining roles. To navigate this complex landscape, it's crucial to explore how genetics can predispose individuals to certain weight-related tendencies while recognizing the powerful influence of lifestyle choices in charting one's weight management journey.

To start, it's important to understand that genetics play a foundational role in determining our body's baseline tendencies. Everyone inherits a unique genetic code that influences myriad physiological aspects, including metabolism, fat storage, and even appetite regulation. Studies have identified specific genes, such as the FTO gene, that can affect body weight by influencing hunger and how the body processes fat. These genetic blueprints might account for why some individuals find it naturally easier to maintain a healthy weight while others struggle despite similar lifestyles.

Nonetheless, genetics aren't destiny. While they establish certain parameters, lifestyle choices are the dynamic variables within these constraints. For instance, two people with the same genetic predisposition might experience vastly different weight outcomes based on their dietary habits, levels of physical activity, and stress management strategies. Effective weight management often involves making conscientious decisions that align with one's genetic predispositions while actively working to mitigate their negative influences.

Consider the role of nutrition. A person might have a genetic predisposition towards gaining weight, particularly with diets high in refined sugars and fats. Awareness of this genetic tendency allows the individual to make informed dietary choices that focus on whole, nutrient-dense foods. This proactive approach can help counteract genetic tendencies and facilitate weight maintenance or loss. It's about crafting a diet that respects and adapts to one's biological inclinations, turning a potential genetic hurdle into a manageable aspect of their lifestyle.

Exercise, too, serves as a powerful counterbalance to genetic influences. Genetic factors might dictate the easy accumulation of fat or predispose an individual to a certain body type. Yet, incorporating regular physical activity can significantly alter this trajectory. Exercise helps improve metabolic health and increases muscle mass, potentially offsetting the metabolic inefficiencies some may be genetically predisposed to. It's the choices we make—like opting for that evening walk or choosing to take the stairs—that empower us to transcend genetic limitations.

Furthermore, consider the impact of mental and emotional health on weight management. While certain genes might affect neurotransmitter levels which, in turn, influence mood and eating behaviors, lifestyle choices play a crucial role. Engaging in mindful eating practices, developing coping mechanisms for stress, and building emotional resilience can help mitigate the effect of such genetic predispositions. The mind-body connection is a potent tool in separating genetic inclination from lifestyle execution, illustrating the power of intentional personal growth and adaptability.

One should also recognize the influence of social and environmental factors. Genetics may wield influence over weight-related tendencies, but an individual's surroundings and social networks often play an equally compelling role. Accessibility to healthy food options, cultural eating norms, and the lifestyle behaviors of friends and family can either reinforce or counteract genetic predispositions. Building a supportive environment might mean creating a kitchen stocked with healthy choices or seeking out a workout buddy to solidify exercise habits. These adaptive strategies highlight how proactive environmental manipulation can counterbalance genetic tendencies.

The journey to understand the interplay between genetic influence and lifestyle choices is as personal as it is complex. It's essential to approach weight management with compassion and flexibility, recognizing that while genetics set the stage, our choices direct the performance. Each step taken in mindful eating, regular exercise, stress management, and social engagement is a testament to the human capacity to adapt and thrive beyond predefined genetic scripts.

This powerful intersection of genetics and lifestyle offers more than just a pathway towards achieving weight-related goals. It serves as a reminder of our inherent agency, illustrating that while we might not write the genetic narrative, we can certainly pen the chapters that determine our health and well-being. Embracing this dual understanding fosters a holistic approach to weight management, one that is informed, intentional, and, ultimately, attainable.

Chapter 2: Nutrition Fundamentals

Welcome to the core of our journey, where food is not the enemy but a valuable ally in your path to sustainable weight loss. Nutrition isn't just about counting calories or cutting carbs; it's about understanding the profound impact of what we consume on our bodies. Whether you're looking to shed a few pounds or embark on a complete lifestyle overhaul, a solid foundation in nutrition is essential.

Let's start by examining macronutrients—carbohydrates, proteins, and fats—the building blocks of our diet. They're not just fuel for our daily activities; they also play a critical role in how our bodies function and thrive. Each macronutrient has a unique purpose. Carbohydrates are the body's primary energy source. Proteins help repair tissues and support muscle growth. Fats, often misunderstood, are crucial for hormone regulation and brain health.

Balancing these macronutrients can feel daunting, but it doesn't have to be. Consider a plate with a healthy diversity of foods: a serving of whole grains like quinoa or brown rice, a portion of lean protein such as chicken or beans, and a healthy fat like avocado or olive oil. This method ensures you're getting the right mix of nutrients to support both your weight loss efforts and overall health.

Meal timing is another component of nutrition that deserves your attention. While the content of your meals is crucial, when you eat also plays a role in weight management. Irregular meal patterns can disrupt your body's natural rhythm, affecting metabolism and energy levels. By establishing a regular eating schedule, you can stabilize blood sugar levels and avoid those tumultuous peaks and valleys that lead to fatigue and cravings.

Intermittent fasting has gained popularity for its potential benefits in improving metabolic health. This approach emphasizes eating within a specific time window and fasting for the remaining hours of the day. For some, this adaptive method can complement weight loss goals. But remember, it's important to listen to your body and find a routine that suits your lifestyle and needs.

Perhaps you're wondering how these principles fit into the bigger picture of weight loss without getting swept up in fad diets or drastic measures. It's all about making informed, thoughtful choices. By being mindful of what and when you eat, you're establishing a sustainable pattern that can lead to lasting success.

It's important to recognize the value of small, incremental changes. When it comes to nutrition, shifting to healthier habits doesn't have to mean overhauling your entire pantry overnight. Start by incorporating more whole foods—vegetables, fruits, whole grains—into your meals. Gradually, these small adjustments will accumulate, leading to significant transformations over time.

No discussion of nutrition would be complete without acknowledging individual differences. What works for one person might not work for another. Factors such as age, sex, activity level, and metabolic health all play a role in determining your nutritional needs. This is why there's no one-size-fits-all solution. Developing an intuitive sense of what fuels your body optimally is the ultimate goal.

Moreover, cultivating a healthy relationship with food is transformative. It's about more than just what's on your plate; it's about appreciating the power of nourishment and the joy of eating. Reject the notion of good and bad foods. Instead, focus on balance and moderation. Give yourself permission to enjoy meals without guilt or restriction, finding satisfaction in every bite.

As you explore the fundamentals of nutrition, remember that this isn't a journey you have to undertake alone. Consider seeking guidance from nutrition professionals who can offer personalized advice tailored to your unique needs. Connect with communities that support your goals, and engage with friends or family who share your vision. Together, these connections can provide you with the encouragement and accountability needed on your path to weight loss success.

In summary, understanding nutrition fundamentals is about empowering yourself to make choices that honor your body's needs. As you continue this journey, be patient and gentle with yourself. With knowledge and perseverance, you're equipped to make lasting changes, leading to a healthier, happier you. Embrace this transformation, armed with the knowledge that nutrition is your powerful tool, not your adversary.

Macronutrients and Their Impact

Understanding macronutrients is like unlocking the code to effective weight loss. At their most basic, macronutrients are the nutrients we need in large amounts to provide energy: carbohydrates, proteins, and fats. Each plays a unique role in our bodies and influences how we feel and function daily. Awareness and balance of these food components can create a profound shift in your approach to eating.

Carbohydrates often get a bad rap in diet culture, yet they're the body's primary energy source. These nutrients are essential for fueling your brain and muscles, especially during physical activities. Carbs come in many forms—simple and complex—but choosing the right type makes all the difference. Emphasizing whole grains, fruits, and vegetables over refined options keeps your energy levels steady and can prevent those infamous midday slumps. Plus, they provide fiber, which aids in digestion and can help you feel full, reducing overall calorie intake. The key is moderation and mindful selection, turning carbs from a foe into a friend in your diet journey.

Protein, on the other hand, is the building block of life. It plays a critical role in repairing tissues, producing important molecules like enzymes and hormones, and supporting immune health. When aiming for weight loss, protein is invaluable due to its ability to keep hunger at bay longer than carbs or fats. Including a variety of protein sources—such as lean meats, fish, beans, and legumes—can help sustain muscle mass during weight loss and boost metabolism. Consider protein as your steady companion for nourishment, strength, and satiety.

Let's not forget about fats, which are often misunderstood. Essential fatty acids found in food are crucial for absorbing vitamins, supporting cell growth, and keeping your body warm. Despite their high calorie content, not all fats are created equal. Unsaturated fats found in avocados, nuts, and olives, for instance, can aid in reducing the risk of heart disease while promoting healthy brain function. Meanwhile, saturated and trans fats, abundant in processed foods, can derail your progress if consumed excessively. The takeaway? Fats are a necessary part of your nutritional spectrum, provided they're consumed in healthy forms and in reasonable amounts.

Balancing macronutrients isn't about adhering to rigid rules; it's about finding what works for your body. Personalizing your ratio of carbohydrates, proteins, and fats can accommodate your lifestyle needs and fitness goals, allowing for a sustainable approach to eating. Does your day include intense workouts or more sedentary desk hours? Tailor your macronutrient intake accordingly to keep energy levels optimal and hunger cues in check. It's also important to note the impact of macronutrients beyond simple calorie counting. They affect hormones that regulate hunger and satiety, like insulin and leptin, directly influencing how we feel after meals. By understanding and respecting these signals, you empower yourself to make smart food choices that align with your body's needs rather than external dietary pressures.

For those striving for effective weight loss, integrating a mixture of carbs, fats, and proteins is akin to assembling a tool kit that's versatile and robust. It's not just about cutting calories; it's about fueling your body so it functions at its best, both physically and mentally. Approach each meal as an opportunity to nourish yourself while being kind and forgiving, knowing that progress is a journey with ups and downs. By mastering the balance of macronutrients, you're laying the groundwork for an eating pattern that not only supports weight loss but also enhances your overall quality of life.

Balancing Carbs, Fats, and Proteins is a cornerstone of understanding how our bodies derive energy and nutrients from the food we consume. When aiming for effective and sustainable weight loss, getting the right balance of these macronutrients is crucial. Let's dive into how to approach this balance, focusing on how each macronutrient contributes to weight loss and overall health.

First, carbohydrates. Often misunderstood and villainized, they are actually our body's preferred energy source. Carbs break down into glucose, which fuels everything from a morning jog to a mind-boggling work meeting. The key isn't to eliminate carbs but to choose complex carbohydrates found in whole grains, fruits, and vegetables. These provide not only energy but also fiber, which aids digestion and keeps hunger at bay. Simple carbohydrates, often found in sugary snacks and white bread, can lead to spikes in blood sugar and should be limited.

Fats, contrary to what many might believe, are not the enemy. They are essential for absorbing vitamins, supporting cell growth, and producing important hormones. The challenge lies in choosing healthy fats, like those found in avocados, nuts, and olive oil, over saturated and trans fats present in fried foods and pastries. Healthy fats satiate us and provide sustained energy, which can prevent overeating. They may also play a role in reducing inflammation and improving heart health.

Proteins are perhaps the most crucial macronutrient when focusing on weight loss due to their role in building and repairing tissues and muscles. Consuming protein-rich foods like lean meats, beans, or tofu at each meal can help maintain muscle mass during weight loss, which is important for keeping metabolism high. Furthermore, protein has a high thermic effect, meaning you burn more calories digesting proteins than carbs or fats, aiding in weight management.

Balancing these macronutrients isn't about strict measures but about moderation and mindfulness. Try to incorporate all three into each meal. For instance, a breakfast of oatmeal topped with fruit and nuts provides a balanced start to the day. It's beneficial to listen to your body; some days you might need more protein after a hard workout, and other days, more carbohydrates to recover from a taxing mental task.

Meal planning and preparation are practical strategies to achieve a balanced intake. By planning meals that incorporate a variety of nutrient-rich foods, you're less likely to reach for unhealthy options. Cooking at home more frequently also helps control portion sizes and ingredient quality, which supports healthier eating habits overall.

It's also important to recognize that individual nutritional needs vary. Factors such as age, gender, lifestyle, and specific health goals can influence the ideal macronutrient balance for someone. Consulting a nutritionist or dietician can provide personalized guidance to navigate these intricacies efficiently.

Moreover, understanding the impact of timing and frequency when balancing macronutrients is crucial. Eating smaller, more frequent meals can help maintain blood sugar levels and prevent energy slumps throughout the day, supporting better food choices and preventing overeating.

Incorporating variety in your diet not only ensures a balance of macronutrients but also prevents monotony, making a balanced diet more sustainable in the long term. It engenders a positive relationship with food, turning meal times into a delightful ritual rather than a chore.

Focusing on nutrient density is also pivotal. Foods rich in vitamins, minerals, and antioxidants provide health benefits beyond their macronutrient content, supporting overall wellness and longevity. Embracing a broad array of colorful fruits and vegetables ensures this nutrient density while keeping meals exciting and satisfying.

Lastly, adopting a balanced macronutrient approach encourages mindful eating practices. Take time to savor the textures and flavors of your meals. Being present during meals reduces the likelihood of overeating and fosters a healthy mind-body connection. When food becomes a source of joy and nourishment rather than stress, the journey to weight loss becomes not just achievable but fulfilling.

In conclusion, while achieving the right balance of carbohydrates, fats, and proteins may appear daunting, it's a manageable process with lasting benefits. By understanding the unique roles and benefits each macronutrient provides, and by making conscious choices, you can support your body's needs and work toward sustainable weight loss goals. Embrace the journey with flexibility and curiosity, knowing that balance leads to not just a trimmer waistline but a healthier, happier life.

The Importance of Meal Timing

Meal timing plays a crucial role in effective and sustainable weight loss. While what you eat holds significant importance, when you eat can also greatly influence your metabolic rate and energy balance. Timing your meals strategically can help in optimizing your metabolism to work in your favor, paving the way for achieving lasting weight management goals.

Eating at regular intervals helps stabilize blood sugar levels and keeps hunger at bay, which can be beneficial in avoiding overeating. This practice of scheduled meals can prevent those unexpected cravings that often lead you to reach for less optimal food choices. By aligning your meal schedule with your body's natural rhythms, also known as your circadian system, you promote not just weight loss but overall well-being.

Intermittent fasting has gained traction as a meal-timing strategy that some find extremely effective. This approach involves designated eating windows and fasting periods, potentially aiding in better appetite control and increased fat burning. Although evidence suggests that intermittent fasting can be a useful tool, it is important to find a pattern that works harmoniously with your lifestyle and needs.

Your body's natural insulin sensitivity is another aspect influenced by meal timing. Typically, insulin sensitivity is higher in the morning, which means your body is more efficient at utilizing nutrients from food. Taking advantage of this by timing your carbohydrate intake earlier in the day can support weight loss efforts. This doesn't mean that late-night snacks are the enemy, but thoughtful adjustments can make a noticeable difference.

Ultimately, integrating meal timing strategies successfully into your life requires patience and attentiveness to your body's signals. Listening to your hunger cues and planning meals that align with both your nutritional needs and lifestyle can empower you to achieve your weight loss goals without resorting to drastic measures. Balance and mindfulness are key for long-term success.

How Meal Schedule Influences Weight Management is a vital consideration within the larger framework of meal timing. It explores how the timing of meals can significantly affect our efforts to manage weight. Meal scheduling is not just about when we eat, but it also relates to consistency and how our bodies respond to the regularity of our eating patterns. By aligning our meals with our circadian rhythms—our internal body clocks—it's possible to optimize weight loss efforts and improve overall health.

When discussing meal schedule, it's crucial to recognize that our bodies are intricate systems designed to operate in cycles. Recent research suggests that eating in sync with our natural circadian rhythms can support metabolic health and weight management. For instance, consuming the majority of calories earlier in the day, when our bodies are more prepared to process energy, may enhance weight loss efforts. This aligns with the saying, "Eat breakfast like a king, lunch like a prince, and dinner like a pauper." Consuming dinner late at night can hinder weight management since it may lead to poorer glucose control and a higher risk of weight gain.

Meal consistency is another key aspect of scheduling that influences weight management. Regular meal patterns can help regulate hunger hormones like ghrelin and leptin, which play a significant role in appetite control and metabolism. Skipping meals or following erratic eating patterns can disrupt these hormones, potentially leading to increased hunger and overeating later. By creating a consistent meal schedule, you're more likely to experience steady energy levels and prevent the temptation of unhealthy snacking.

Consider the evidence supporting a structured meal schedule. Studies have shown that individuals who maintain regular eating times often have better control over their weight compared to those with irregular meal patterns. This regularity helps to set expectations for the body, enabling it to optimize the digestion and absorption of nutrients more effectively. Moreover, having a predictable meal schedule can reduce stress around mealtimes, contributing to healthier eating habits overall.

Strategically planning meals around activity levels can also stay beneficial. Consuming a balanced meal post-exercise can ensure that your body has the nutrients it needs to recover and build muscle efficiently. This, in turn, aids in boosting your metabolism, an essential factor in weight management. Aligning meal times with your daily energy expenditure supports effective weight management by ensuring that you're fueling your body when it needs energy most, rather than when it's winding down for the day.

It's not just about what and when you eat, but about how your body utilizes that fuel. Understanding the science of meal timing provides an opportunity to make informed decisions about when to consume different types of macronutrients. For example, carbohydrates might be best consumed earlier in the day when the body can use that glucose effectively for energy needs, while proteins are beneficial post-exercise for muscle repair and growth.

The psychological aspect of meal scheduling shouldn't be overlooked either. Having a reliable eating schedule can reduce anxiety and enhance emotional well-being by providing a framework in which food is consumed. This can ultimately lower the risk of stress-induced eating, a common barrier to successful weight management. Knowing when your next meal is can offer peace of mind and help regulate portions and choices more effectively.

While adopting a structured meal schedule, it is important to listen to your body's signals. Intuitive eating—being attuned to your body's hunger and fullness cues—is a skill that can be developed over time by those maintaining a consistent eating schedule. This empowers individuals to differentiate between emotional and physical hunger, aiding in making mindful choices that align with their weight loss goals.

Importantly, meal scheduling should remain flexible enough to accommodate social interactions and personal preferences. The goal isn't to rigidly adhere to a clock but to find a sustainable pattern that aligns with your lifestyle, making weight management a more harmonious part of daily life. It's about creating a routine that's adaptable yet consistent enough to support metabolic rhythm and energy levels.

As you consider how to implement meal scheduling into your life, keep in mind that it's an ongoing process. Experimenting with different meal times and observing how your body responds can provide valuable insights. An individualized approach is key—everyone's body is unique, and what works for one person may not be ideal for another. Patience and persistence will yield the best outcomes as you find what aligns with your body's natural cycles.

In conclusion, the impact of meal scheduling on weight management emphasizes the significance of regularity and alignment with our body's natural rhythms. By prioritizing when we eat alongside what we eat, we can create a supportive environment for our metabolism and overall health. In doing so, we empower ourselves to achieve and maintain our weight loss goals in a sustainable and fulfilling manner.

Chapter 3: Debunking Diet Myths

In the world of weight loss, myths float around like clouds, ever-shifting but always present. They often promise quick solutions but deliver little more than confusion and disappointment. Let's shine a light on these misconceptions and explore why they often do more harm than good.

One major myth that needs debunking is the notion that low-carb diets are the magic bullet for weight loss. Carbohydrates have long been pegged as the culprit for weight gain. However, the truth is more nuanced. While it's true that reducing refined carbs can support weight loss, eliminating carbs altogether can deprive your body of essential nutrients. Complex carbohydrates found in whole grains, vegetables, and legumes are vital sources of energy. Instead of cutting out carbs entirely, a more balanced approach ensures that you're fueling your body effectively without excessive calorie intake.

Fad diets are another set of myths dressed in flashy packaging. They often make grandiose claims of shedding pounds within days. Diets like these come and go, leaving a trail of frustrated followers in their wake. The problem lies in their unsustainable nature. They often impose severe restrictions that are hard to maintain long-term. Our bodies thrive on consistency and balance, not on drastic changes. By understanding the root cause of weight gain, both dietary and lifestyle, we can create sustainable habits rather than chasing temporary fixes.

Let's also talk about the idea that all calories are created equal. This simplification ignores the complex ways different foods affect our bodies. For instance, 100 calories of candy act very differently from 100 calories of vegetables. Nutrient density matters, as does how your body processes different kinds of foods. Foods rich in fiber and protein not only fill you up longer but also rev up your metabolism. Recognizing that the quality of calories is as important as the quantity can transform your approach to eating.

Then there's the misconception that skipping meals can speed up weight loss. Skipping meals generally leads to overeating later on and disrupts your body's hunger cues. Maintaining a regular eating pattern supports metabolic efficiency and helps regulate insulin levels. Consistent, smaller meals can maintain your energy levels throughout the day, keeping you focused and active.

Despite the proliferation of myths, the path to effective weight loss doesn't have to be shrouded in mystery. It's a journey of understanding and action. By lifting the veil on false promises, you gain the freedom to make informed choices. Choose to fuel your body with nutritious foods, embrace physical activity, and develop habits that fit your lifestyle. Empowerment in your weight loss journey comes from knowledge and understanding. Facts over flash, consistency over quick fixes. As each myth is debunked, you're armed with the insight needed to carve out your own unique path to lasting success. With a clear mind and a commitment to truth, every step you take brings you closer to your goals.

The Truth About Low-Carb Diets

Low-carb diets have swept through the nutritional landscape like a whirlwind, sparking passionate debates and countless transformations. As you dive into the intricacies of weight loss, it's crucial to see beyond the aura that surrounds low-carb eating plans and focus on their real potential and limitations.

The appeal of low-carb diets, like Atkins and keto, often lies in their promise of rapid weight loss. By significantly reducing carbohydrate intake, these diets encourage your body to tap into its fat stores for energy, leading to what's known as ketosis. This process can indeed result in noticeable weight loss in the short term. However, it's important to recognize that initial weight loss often stems more from water loss than fat. Carbohydrates store water in the body, so cutting them out can lead to quick, but sometimes misleading, results. While this drop on the scale can be motivating, it doesn't necessarily equate to sustainable fat loss.

Moreover, the human body is amazingly adaptable, which means it can adjust to different dietary conditions. While ketosis can be an effective means for shedding pounds, there's a catch: maintaining such a restrictive diet long-term can be challenging for many. One of the key criticisms of low-carb diets is their difficulty in adherence. Carbs, especially complex ones like whole grains and legumes, are often deeply ingrained in cultural and social eating practices, making their exclusion a potential pitfall for long-term success.

The world of nutrition is full of seeming contradictions. While some shun carbs, it's worth recognizing that not all carbohydrates are created equal. The blanket demonization of carbs ignores the benefits of whole, fiber-rich sources. These contain essential nutrients that our bodies need to function optimally. Whole grains, for instance, offer fiber, which is crucial for gut health and can even aid in weight management by promoting a feeling of fullness. In contrast, refined carbs, like white bread and pastries, provide little nutritional value and can spike blood sugar levels, often leading to cravings and overeating.

There's also the enjoyable aspect of food that many low-carb diets challenge. Sharing a pasta dish with friends or having a slice of birthday cake can be integral to social interactions and personal enjoyment. Cutting carbs entirely might complicate these everyday experiences, leading to a sense of isolation or deprivation. The key is mindfulness and moderation, rather than outright exclusion.

Consider the psychological impact of restricting a major food group like carbohydrates. Often, creating a food environment characterized by scarcity can trigger heightened desires and even binges. The cycle of restriction and overindulgence can be emotionally taxing and might derail the weight loss journey. Building a sustainable and balanced approach often requires rethinking not just what we eat, but how we perceive food.

A strategy that often emerges as more sustainable is the integration of mindful eating habits, focusing on balance and building a positive relationship with all macro-nutrients, including carbohydrates. It's crucial to find a dietary approach that fits one's lifestyle and preferences. Achieving this balance could be the pivotal factor in not only losing weight but keeping it off.

Ultimately, the truth about low-carb diets is not about placing them on a pedestal or condemning them. It's about understanding their strengths and the specific scenarios where they might be beneficial. It's also about recognizing their limitations and knowing when flexibility and balance offer a more sustainable path. Nutrition is deeply personal, and the best approach is the one that aligns with your life and goals, allowing you to thrive physically and emotionally. Empower yourself with knowledge, experiment within safe boundaries, and choose a path that harmonizes with your unique needs and lifestyle.

Carb Myths and Realities can easily trip us up on our journey to effective weight loss. For years, there's been a cloud of mystery around carbohydrates. Are they the enemy, or do they have a place in our diets? Many people embark on low-carb diets expecting dramatic results, only to find themselves caught in a cycle of misinformation and confusion. It's time we untangle the myths from the facts, providing a clearer picture of what carbohydrates really mean for our health.

One of the most prevalent myths is that all carbs lead to weight gain. In reality, not all carbs are created equal. Whole grains, fruits, and vegetables contain complex carbohydrates that provide essential nutrients and energy. Our bodies rely on these carbs for fuel, particularly for brain function and physical activity. Eliminating them completely can deprive the body of key nutrients and lead to fatigue and digestive issues.

Conversely, refined carbs, found in sugary cereals, sodas, and white bread, offer little nutritional benefit and can indeed lead to weight gain if consumed excessively. It's important to differentiate the sources of our carbohydrates. Focusing on quality over quantity can help maintain a balanced diet without unnecessary sacrifice. By choosing complex carbs, we can keep energy levels steady and avoid the crashes that often accompany diets high in refined sugars.

Another misconception is that going low-carb delivers instant and sustainable weight loss. While it's true that reducing carbs can lead to quick initial losses, often due to water weight and glycogen depletion, the long-term sustainability is questionable. Many people find low-carb diets challenging to maintain, leading to yo-yo dieting effects, where weight is lost and regained repeatedly. Long-term success often requires a balanced approach, not drastic elimination.

There's also the notion that low-carb diets are the best for everyone. We must acknowledge individual differences in metabolism and lifestyle when considering such diets. Some people thrive on lower carbs due to metabolic variations, while others may feel sluggish and deprived. Personalization is key when navigating these waters. What works for one person might not yield the same results for another. Listening to your body and adjusting accordingly can make all the difference.

Low-carb diets have been hailed for promoting weight loss by triggering a state of ketosis, where the body burns fat instead of carbs for energy. However, maintaining ketosis consistently is difficult, and many people struggle with dietary restrictions and potential nutrient deficiencies. Moreover, there's no magic bullet in weight loss, and focusing solely on carbs without considering overall caloric balance, activity levels, and nutritional variety can limit success.

It's worth noting that carbs play a vital role in athletic performance. For athletes and physically active individuals, carbs are crucial for sustaining energy levels and enhancing recovery. It's a myth that cutting them completely yields better performance. Instead, a proper balance can boost endurance and reduce fatigue, affirming that carbs do have a legitimate place in a performance-oriented diet.

Moreover, the demonization of carbs often overlooks the benefits of fiber-rich foods. These complex carbohydrates improve digestion, promote satiety, and aid in the regulation of blood sugar levels. Diets that exclude these foods may inadvertently increase hunger and make weight management more challenging. Emphasizing fiber intake can support a more sustainable approach to eating. Focusing on whole foods ensures a diet rich in necessary nutrients.

Examining cultural dietary patterns also highlights carb inconsistencies. Various cultures around the world thrive on diets high in carbohydrates, such as the Mediterranean or Okinawan diets, known for supporting longevity and health. These diets emphasize the right kinds of carbs, combined with healthy fats and proteins, proving that a blanket low-carb approach isn't universally applicable. Adopting a mindful approach to carbohydrates encourages a balanced exchange of nutrients.

Finally, the fear of carbs often leads to the neglect of important body signals. Hunger cues are natural and ignoring them due to strict dietary rules can result in overeating later on. Instead of fighting against our bodies, we should learn to attune to their needs. Respecting hunger and fullness cues while choosing nourishing carbs can guide healthier eating patterns. Balance becomes more achievable when we're mentally tuned into the body's signals.

Understanding carb myths and realities empowers people to make informed dietary decisions. It's about balance, quality, and personalization, rather than extreme exclusion. When we debunk dieting myths, we're free to construct diets that are nourishing and sustainable. Armed with knowledge, the path to weight loss becomes less about restriction and more about mindful choices that honor our body's true needs.

Fad Diets Examined

In the world of dieting, fads come and go like tides, often leaving people feeling confused and defeated. These trendy diets promise rapid weight loss and often boast of magical solutions, yet they rarely deliver lasting results. One of the biggest pitfalls of fad diets is their inability to offer sustainable change. They're usually so restrictive—cutting out entire food groups or demanding adherence to extreme calorie counts—that they become impossible to maintain over time.

People are drawn to the allure of quick fixes, and it's understandable. In a society that values instant gratification, the thought of shedding pounds fast is very tempting. But here's the reality: fad diets offer a "quick win" that's often followed by a not-so-quick rebound. You lose weight rapidly, only to gain it back, sometimes with extra pounds tagging along. This is not only discouraging but can also be damaging to your overall health. Let's consider some common fad diets. There's the cabbage soup diet, the grapefruit diet, and even more extreme options like the tapeworm diet—yes, you read that right. Such diets tend to focus narrowly on one type of food or strategy, neglecting the complete nutritional needs of the body. This not only prevents long-term weight maintenance but can lead to nutrient deficiencies and metabolic disruptions.

The sell is always the same: neat before-and-after photos, tantalizingly simple rules, and testimonials that promise life-changing results. But what those glamorous ads won't tell you is that long-term adherence is low. People often revert to their old eating habits, feeling defeated by the diet's unsustainable nature. The cycle of losing and regaining weight—also known as yo-yo dieting—has its own risks, including cardiovascular complications and muscle loss.

A genuinely effective weight management plan should feel less like a punishment and more like a supportive partnership. Building a diet that's balanced, flexible, and compassionate holds the key to effective, long-lasting change. You deserve to eat meals that nourish both your body and spirit, without the guilt or stress that accompanies so many fad diets. It's about creating a harmonious relationship with food, where you listen to your body's needs rather than fighting against them.

So, why do these diets still capture our attention? Maybe because they're marketed as revolutionary or because they promise results without requiring a thorough lifestyle change. But transforming your body and health for the long haul won't come from a fad. It requires patience, learning, and a dash of self-compassion. Trade the impatience for a strategy rooted in self-discovery and education. That's how we make progress in a way that's meaningful and sustainable.

Taking a step back from the allure of quick fixes can feel daunting, but it's a step towards empowerment. Challenge yourself to question the promises of those fad diets and consider what truly nourishes your body and soul. In seeking effective and sustainable weight loss, remember that true transformation doesn't come with a rapid fix, but with gradual, enduring changes you can live with—and thrive with—for a lifetime.

Why Trendy Diets Fail Long-term In our pursuit of rapid weight loss, it's easy to be lured by the promises of trendy diets. They're alluringly packaged, supported by celebrity endorsements, and promise astounding results in impossibly short timeframes. However, when we peel back the glossy exterior, the fundamental flaw becomes evident: these diets aren't designed for longevity. They often ignore the very principles that foster lasting change, leaving individuals disenchanted and back at square one.

Trendy diets often operate on a principle of restriction. Whether it's eliminating entire food groups, drastically cutting calories, or mandating specific eating windows, these diets create a short-term illusion of success. Rapid weight loss can occur, but it's rarely sustainable. The human body has evolved over millennia to adapt in environments of scarcity and abundance, so when you restrict essential nutrients or energy, it triggers survival mechanisms that can lead to rebound weight gain once the diet's over.

Moreover, these diets can negatively impact both physical and mental health. Physically, extreme dietary restrictions can deprive the body of vital nutrients necessary for maintaining health and vitality. This deprivation can manifest as fatigue, weakened immunity, and even more severe health complications over time. Mentally, the rigidity and monotony of trendy diets can create an unhealthy relationship with food, fostering anxiety, guilt, and a cycle of yo-yo dieting that can be difficult to break.

Another critical factor in the failure of trendy diets is the lack of personalization. Weight management is profoundly personal, intertwining genetic makeup, lifestyle, emotional health, and more. A one-size-fits-all approach often disregards these complexities. What works for one person may not work for another, and prescribed cookie-cutter diets often neglect to account for individual needs, preferences, and lifestyle constraints. These omissions are significant roadblocks to creating a sustainable eating pattern.

Behavioral psychology also plays a pivotal role here. Humans are creatures of habit, and changing those habits requires intention and time, along with a deep understanding of one's motivations and triggers. Fad diets often promise quick results, which undermine the psychological perseverance needed for a true lifestyle transformation. When the novelty wears off or when expectations aren't met as projected, motivation wanes, often leading individuals back to old habits.

Consider the impact on social and cultural aspects of eating. Food is intrinsically tied to culture, tradition, and connection. Trendy diets can isolate individuals from their social circles, as they can't participate in communal meals or cultural celebrations without breaking their diet's strict rules. This isolation can contribute to feelings of exclusion and an eventual rejection of the dieting principles themselves.

It's also crucial to acknowledge how these diets often fail to teach essential skills for maintaining weight loss. Strategies for coping with emotional eating, understanding hunger signals, and making informed food choices are rarely part of the equation. Without these skills, individuals may find themselves lost and vulnerable to weight regain once they return to their usual routines.

So, how can one escape the siren call of trendy diets and embrace a path to lasting weight loss? First, it's important to focus on building a foundation of healthy habits rather than looking for quick fixes. This means viewing weight loss as a journey rather than a destination and embracing small, incremental changes that can be maintained for life.

Integrating balanced eating with regular activity and nurturing mental well-being can form a holistic approach that stands the test of time.

Educational empowerment is another key piece. Learning about the body's nutritional needs, how different foods affect energy levels, mood, and overall health, and how to make delicious, healthy meals can transform the diet from a fleeting trend to a sustainable lifestyle. Additionally, surrounding oneself with support from friends, family, or professionals who align with healthy living goals can provide motivation and accountability, paving the way for success when challenges arise.

The allure of trendy diets may never fully disappear, but understanding why they fail long-term equips us with the knowledge to make more informed, compassionate choices for our bodies. As we embrace this shift, we begin to view eating not merely as a means to an end but as an integral, cherished component of a balanced and fulfilling life.

Chapter 4: Exercise Essentials for Weight Loss

Embarking on a weight loss journey brings you face-to-face with the pivotal role of exercise. It's not just about torching calories—exercise transforms you in ways far beyond the numbers on a scale. While it's easy to envision exercise as grueling hours on a treadmill, the essence of a successful workout regimen lies in balance, sustainability, and joy.

Cardio workouts frequently dominate the conversation when discussing exercise for weight loss. These workouts, ranging from brisk walks to high-intensity interval training (HIIT), are highly effective for revving up the heart rate and increasing energy expenditure. When you elevate the heart rate during exercise, your body taps into stored fat as fuel, making cardio an essential element in shedding extra pounds. But remember, it's not about pushing yourself to the brink; it's about finding a rhythm and routine that suits your lifestyle and keeps you motivated. Start slow, perhaps with a ten-minute daily walk, and gradually increase intensity and duration as confidence builds.

While cardio is vital, strength training is another critical piece of the weight loss puzzle. There's a common misconception that strength training is solely for those looking to bulk up. On the contrary, building muscle accelerates metabolism, helping you burn more calories even while at rest. Lifting weights or engaging in bodyweight exercises like push-ups and squats does more than sculpt your physique; it empowers you to become a calorie-burning powerhouse. Muscle tissue is metabolically active, meaning that the more muscle you have, the more energy your body expends.

Integration of both cardio and strength training maximizes results. A routine that combines the sweat-inducing sprints of cardio sessions with muscle-strengthening lifts creates a balanced, effective approach to weight loss. Variety keeps things engaging—the body thrives on change. When exercise becomes monotonous, stagnation occurs, and motivation wanes. Keep things fresh by incorporating new activities such as cycling, swimming, or yoga, which not only invigorate the body but also rejuvenate the mind.

Exercise also has profound effects on mental health, an often-overlooked aspect of the weight loss journey. Physical activity releases endorphins, known as the brain's natural mood enhancers. These chemicals foster a feeling of well-being and positivity, reducing stress and lowering perceptions of fatigue. When exercise becomes a regular part of your routine, you tap into reservoirs of new energy, resilience, and focus, transforming challenges into opportunities for growth.

For those battling the intricacies of weight loss, accountability can be a game-changer. Find a workout buddy or engage in group classes to stay committed to your routine. There's strength in numbers, and exercising in a community fosters camaraderie and support that can propel you through moments of doubt or fatigue. People around you can offer the encouragement you need to push through hurdles or simply be there as you both enjoy the shared journey.

An often underestimated aspect of exercise is flexibility and balance. Workouts should be designed to improve these areas, contributing to overall fitness and well-being. Balance exercises like Tai Chi or Pilates help enhance your core strength and stability, reducing the risk of injury. Flexibility routines, such as regular stretching or yoga, aid in maintaining joint health and muscle function, which is crucial as you up your exercise game. Ultimately, the key to incorporating exercise into your weight loss strategy lies in personalizing your plan. Set realistic goals that align with your lifestyle, interests, and schedule. If mornings are your time of peace, try an early jog. If evenings suit you better, wind down with an evening spin class. The crucial part is consistency, not perfection. Celebrate each small victory—whether it's adding five more push-ups to your set or jogging an extra block—and let these successes motivate you toward bigger milestones. In your journey, it's easy to get caught up in the pursuit of visible results, but consider the invisible changes happening within. Your heart is getting stronger, your stamina is increasing, and you are acquiring tools for stress relief and improved mental health. Each step, lift, and stretch brings you closer to a healthier, happier you. Embrace the process, find joy in movement, and let exercise be the catalyst that sparks transformation and sustains your path to lasting weight loss.

The Science of Cardio Workouts

When it comes to weight loss, cardio workouts often take center stage, and with good reason. Cardio, short for cardiovascular exercise, engages your heart and circulatory system, boosting your metabolism and burning calories in the process. For many, the journey to a healthier weight begins with the simple act of raising their heart rate. Cardio exercises are not just about losing weight; they are about building a robust, healthier body from the inside out.

Cardio encompasses a wide range of activities, from brisk walking and cycling to swimming and dancing. All of these exercises share one common feature: they increase your heart rate. This increased heart rate encourages your body to burn stored energy, which primarily comes from carbohydrates and fats. The science is clear: when you engage in regular cardio workouts, your body becomes more efficient at using these energy sources, which in turn facilitates weight loss. But beyond this, cardio workouts also trigger the release of endorphins, those feel-good hormones that can transform exercise from a chore into a source of joy and stress relief.

The key to maximizing the benefits of cardio workouts lies in understanding how they interact with your body's metabolic processes. During these exercises, your body consumes oxygen to convert stored fats and carbohydrates into energy. This increased energy expenditure can lead to a calorie deficit, which is crucial for weight loss. The more intense your cardio session, the more calories you're likely to burn. However, it's not just about going all out. Finding the right balance and rhythm for your body can help you maintain a consistent routine while avoiding burnout.

One of the most compelling aspects of cardio workouts is their versatility. They can be tailored to fit any lifestyle, offering low-impact options like walking and swimming for beginners, as well as high-intensity interval training (HIIT) for those seeking a challenge. HIIT, in particular, has gained popularity due to its efficiency and effectiveness. This type of training mixes short bursts of intense activity with periods of rest or lower-intensity exercise, boosting your metabolism long after the workout ends through a process known as excess post-exercise oxygen consumption (EPOC).

Diversity is another advantage of cardio workouts. Whether it's a dance class, a long run through the park, or a cycling session, the variety keeps you engaged and motivated. It's crucial, however, to listen to your body. As much as cardio can be a powerful tool in achieving weight loss goals, overexertion can lead to injuries or fatigue. Start with what feels comfortable and gradually increase intensity as your fitness level improves. This gradual progression not only helps in preventing injuries but also aids in forming a sustainable routine that aligns with your long-term weight loss goals.

Moreover, the benefits of cardio go beyond just weight loss. Regular aerobic activity strengthens your heart and lungs, reduces the risk of chronic diseases such as hypertension and diabetes, and enhances your overall well-being. It's a holistic practice that not only supports you in shedding pounds but also contributes to a healthier, more vibrant life. Understanding how cardio fits into your weight loss journey can empower you to make informed choices about your fitness routine. Whether it's a morning jog or an afternoon swim, these activities serve as crucial components of a balanced lifestyle. As you incorporate cardio into your regimen, remember why you started and celebrate the small victories along the way. It's not just about the numbers on the scale; it's about embracing a more active and fulfilling life.

Ultimately, the science of cardio workouts lies in their ability to engage your heart, elevate your spirits, and transform your body. By integrating these exercises into your daily routine, you're not only working toward a healthier weight but also investing in a longer, more vibrant life. As you move forward, let each step and heartbeat remind you that you're capable of achieving your goals, one cardio session at a time.

Optimizing Cardio for Fat Loss involves understanding the nuanced relationship between cardio workouts and their effectiveness in shedding excess weight. When it comes to weight loss, there's a common misconception that simply hitting the treadmill for hours on end will melt the pounds away. But the science of cardio workouts reveals a more strategic approach is needed. Cardio, short for cardiovascular exercise, boosts the heart rate and increases energy expenditure, crucial for fat loss. However, the key lies in optimizing these workouts to maximize fat burning while maintaining healthy muscle mass, aligning with your weight loss goals.

It's paramount to understand that the body taps into different energy sources depending on the intensity and duration of exercise. During low to moderate-intensity cardiovascular activities, the body primarily burns fat as its energy source. For individuals just beginning their weight loss journey, starting with moderate-intensity exercises like brisk walking, cycling, or swimming can optimize fat burning while being gentle on the joints and muscles. These activities not only improve cardiovascular health but also establish a sustainable routine that can be gradually intensified.

Interval training has surged in popularity and for good reasons. It's a catalyst for improved fat loss, offering more effective results in less time. High-Intensity Interval Training (HIIT), characterized by bursts of high-intensity exercise followed by rest or low-intensity recovery, has been shown to significantly elevate the metabolic rate, not just during the workout but for hours after completion. This is due to an effect known as excess post-exercise oxygen consumption (EPOC). By incorporating HIIT into a regular exercise regimen, individuals can reap more of the fat-burning benefits without spending excessive time in the gym.

However, caution is advised when engaging in high-intensity workouts, especially for beginners. Starting with lower intensity intervals can help avoid injury and accommodate one's current fitness level. Over time, as fitness improves, the intensity and duration of the high-effort segments can be increased.

Moreover, personalization in cardio workouts is critical for amplifying fat loss. What works for one person might not be ideal for another, and this is where individual preferences and body responses should guide the exercise plan. Tracking progress through tools like heart rate monitors or fitness apps can provide valuable insights. Monitoring how your body reacts to different types of cardio can help tailor your approach, ensuring it remains effective and enjoyable. This keeps motivation high and boredom at bay.

Nutritional support acts as the bedrock to any cardio regimen aimed at fat loss. Exercising on an empty stomach, often touted as "fasted cardio," can push the body to use fat as a primary energy source. However, its efficiency varies among individuals. Some may perform better with a small pre-workout snack to prevent fatigue. Experimentation and listening to one's body will determine what works best. Post-workout nutrition also comes into play, where consuming a mix of proteins and carbohydrates can aid recovery and muscle preservation.

Consistency trumps everything when optimizing cardio for fat loss. Short bursts of motivation must transform into long-term habits. Scheduling regular cardio sessions, similar to any important meeting, prevents the classic pitfall of inconsistent efforts that yield little results. It's the accumulation of these sessions over time, compounded by strategic intensity variations, that transform an active lifestyle into an effective weight loss tool.

For those struggling to maintain interest, creativity in cardio choices can reignite motivation. Alternatives to traditional cardio like dance, sports, or team-based activities can introduce a fun element, making workouts feel less like drudgery and more like recreation. Such variations not only engage different muscle groups but also support mental health, keeping stress levels in check.

Lastly, integrating rest and recovery is fundamental. Cardio exercises can place a substantial load on the cardiovascular system and muscles. Balancing effort with adequate recovery prevents burnout and injuries, ultimately keeping one on track toward fat loss goals. Active recovery, incorporating light activities such as yoga or stretching, can complement the rest days without losing momentum.

In summary, optimizing cardio for fat loss requires a multifaceted approach. It requires aligning personal interests with scientific insights into how different cardio regimes affect the body's fat-burning capabilities. By customizing workouts, adjusting intensity, and supporting efforts with proper nutrition and recovery, individuals can harness cardio exercises' full potential to not only lose weight but keep it off sustainably. The journey isn't about quick fixes, but rather creating a lifestyle where physical activity becomes an enjoyable and integral part of everyday life.

Strength Training Benefits

When it comes to weight loss, most people instinctively think of long cardio sessions that leave them drenched in sweat. While cardio undoubtedly has its place in a balanced routine, strength training often holds the key to unlocking your body's potential in the weight loss journey. Surprisingly, lifting weights may do as much good—if not more—for those seeking sustainable change. In this section, we'll uncover the multi-faceted benefits of strength training and how it can transform both your body and mind.

Strength training is not just about building bulging muscles. It's about enhancing your body's natural ability to burn fat more efficiently. Engaging in regular resistance exercises leads to the development of lean muscle mass. Muscle tissue is metabolically active, meaning it requires energy to maintain, even at rest. This elevated energy demand results in a higher resting metabolic rate, which helps increase the number of calories burned throughout the day. Simply put, the more muscle you have, the more calories your body torches, setting the stage for effective weight management.

Moreover, there's a profound psychological component that comes with strength training. As you gradually lift heavier weights and push your boundaries, your confidence blossoms. There's something inherently empowering about lifting weights, and that empowerment can spill over into other aspects of life. It's not just about gaining physical strength; it's about building strength in character, resilience, and determination.

As we age, we naturally lose muscle mass— a process known as sarcopenia. This loss is often accompanied by a decrease in metabolism, posing challenges for maintaining a healthy weight. Strength training offers a way to counteract this age-related decline. By prioritizing resistance exercises in your fitness routine, you actively combat muscle loss, supporting both your metabolism and overall functionality as the years pass.

The benefits stretch beyond weight loss, too. Participation in regular strength training can improve bone density, which becomes increasingly important as we age. Enhanced bone density reduces the risk of fractures and osteoporosis, particularly crucial for women post-menopause when bone density naturally decreases. Through resistance exercises, you promote bone health, providing an invaluable safeguard for the future.

For those worried about dedicating hours to the gym, fear not. Strength training is remarkably flexible and time-efficient. Short, intense sessions can have a high impact when consistently incorporated into your routine. Whether you're using bodyweight exercises, free weights, or resistance machines, you can tailor the workouts to fit your lifestyle and goals. This flexibility ensures that you're less likely to grow bored or overwhelmed, making it easier to stick with your fitness journey.

An often underrated aspect of strength training is its role in injury prevention. By strengthening muscles, tendons, and ligaments, you provide better support for your joints, reducing the likelihood of injuries. It enhances balance and coordination, critical elements in maintaining an active and fulfilling lifestyle. For sports enthusiasts, this can mean fewer setbacks and more time enjoying the activities you love.

Beyond the physical realm, strength training offers mental health benefits that are equally compelling. Exercise, particularly weight training, triggers the release of endorphins, the body's natural mood elevators. This endorphin rush can reduce stress, alleviate symptoms of anxiety, and combat depression. When you feel good mentally, you're more likely to make healthier choices, reinforcing a positive cycle in your weight loss journey.

Speaking of mental health, let's touch on the mental discipline strength training instills. The focus required to perform a lift with proper form demands attention and mindfulness. This practice not only improves your workouts but can translate into other domains of life, strengthening your ability to concentrate and tackle problems with clarity.

Social benefits exist, too. Whether you join a strength training class or simply chat with others at the gym, there's a camaraderie in the shared pursuit of fitness goals. This support network can motivate you to keep progressing, offer a seasoned perspective, and even elevate your enjoyment of strength training.

It's important to note that embarking on strength training doesn't necessitate giving up other forms of exercise. Instead, consider integrating it into a well-rounded fitness regimen that includes cardiovascular workouts and flexibility exercises. Each element has its role, together promoting improved physical health and well-being.

Lastly, a common myth to dispel—strength training won't make you bulky overnight. Women, in particular, might fear looking too muscular, but achieving significant muscle mass requires specialized training and dietary modifications. The goal here is not to transform overnight but to harness the benefits of muscle development in a balanced, realistic way.

Incorporating strength training into your weight loss plan doesn't just reshape your physique; it reshapes your mindset, amplifying both physical and mental resilience. With commitment and consistency, you're not merely lifting weights; you're lifting the weight of self-imposed limitations, inching closer to the healthiest, most empowered version of yourself.

Building Muscle to Boost Metabolism isn't just about sculpting a physique that turns heads—though that's a nice side effect—it's about creating a solid foundation for effective and sustainable weight loss. When we think of strength training, it's easy to imagine rows of treadmills and racks of free weights. Yet, the real magic happens in how this form of exercise transforms not just our bodies, but also our metabolism, turning it into a more efficient calorie-burning machine.

First, let's dive into the mechanics. When you engage in strength training, you're effectively tearing down muscle fibers. The body, in its adaptive brilliance, repairs these tiny tears stronger than before, a process known as muscle hypertrophy. This muscle-building not only enhances physical strength but also significantly boosts your resting metabolic rate (RMR). Each pound of muscle burns more calories than its fat counterpart, even when you're lounging around watching your favorite show. Think of muscle as the engine of a high-performance car, revving up your metabolism.

Here's why this matters on a practical level: a higher RMR means you're effectively burning more calories throughout the day—during workouts, rest, and even sleep. The calorie deficit needed for weight loss becomes more attainable without requiring drastic dietary restrictions or hours spent on cardio machines. This metabolic boost presents a more realistic and sustainable strategy for shedding those unwanted pounds. It's not just about working harder; it's about letting your body work smarter for you.

Moreover, strength training does more than just impact your metabolism. It plays a critical role in maintaining bone density, which is particularly beneficial as we age. By stimulating bones through weight-bearing activity, you reduce the risk of osteoporosis and other age-related degenerative conditions. Enhanced muscle mass also supports joint stability and flexibility, creating a buffer against injuries. This makes it an ideal choice for any age group seeking to lose weight without risking their mobility.

Beyond the physical benefits, there's a substantial mental gain. Engaging in strength routines can build confidence, resilience, and a sense of achievement. As you watch your capabilities grow and your body transform, it sparks a mental shift towards a more positive self-image. This mental boost can be crucial in maintaining motivation and commitment to your weight loss journey.

Integrating regular strength training into your routine doesn't have to be daunting. Start small by incorporating bodyweight exercises like squats, push-ups, and lunges, which are incredibly effective and don't require any equipment. As you gain confidence and strength, consider using resistance bands, free weights, or gym machines. Remember, consistency trumps intensity. It's about gradual progression and finding a rhythm that suits your lifestyle.

It's worth mentioning the role of recovery. As muscles grow and metabolism rises, so does your need for adequate rest. Muscles develop during periods of rest and recovery—not during workouts. Ensure that your regimen includes rest days and quality sleep, allowing your body to repair and build effectively. Hydration and nutrition also play supportive roles, aiding in recovery and optimizing muscle growth.

Attempting to lose weight through exercise demands a keen balance between cardio and strength training. While cardio exercises are excellent for immediate calorie burning, it is the strength training that lays down the groundwork for long-term metabolism

Emotional Eating Uncovered

Emotional eating is a complex dance between mind and body. Often, we find ourselves reaching for comfort food not because we're hungry but because we're trying to fill an emotional void. Perhaps it's stress from work, a fight with a loved one, or just the loneliness of a quiet evening. The immediate gratification from eating can seem like a balm for our emotions, yet it's typically fleeting, leaving us with guilt instead of comfort.

It's crucial to understand that emotional eating is not a sign of weakness. Instead, it's a learned response that can be unlearned. Emotional eating isn't about the food; it's about what's beneath the surface. Our culture often encourages a "treat yourself" mentality, which makes it all the more challenging to spot these patterns. Recognizing when you're eating for emotions rather than hunger is the first step toward reclaiming control.

Think of emotional eating as an iceberg. What you're aware of is just the tip—what's driving it is hidden beneath the water. These drivers might be boredom, fatigue, anxiety, or even happiness. The solution involves unveiling these emotions, understanding them, and developing new, healthier coping strategies. Perhaps it's a walk outside, a few moments of deep breathing, or even a conversation with a friend.

Change isn't instantaneous. Developing a new relationship with food takes time and patience. One practical approach is keeping a food and mood journal. By associating certain foods with particular emotions, you start to notice patterns. This awareness is crucial—it empowers you to make mindful decisions about when and why you eat. It's not about restriction but about choice.

Building a supportive environment also plays a critical role in tackling emotional eating. Share your journey with those close to you. You'd be surprised how discussing your struggles with emotional eating with a friend or family member can relieve some of the pressure. When you bring these issues to light, they lose some of their power over you.

Ultimately, conquering emotional eating is about embracing self-compassion. Be gentle with yourself as you explore these behaviors. You're likely to have setbacks, but these are growth opportunities rather than failures. Every step towards understanding your emotional eating habits nudges you closer to a healthier, more balanced life.

Remember, your journey is your own. You have the tools within you to make meaningful change. By nurturing a more intuitive relationship with food and emotions, you'll not only contribute to your weight loss goals but also foster a healthier, more fulfilling lifestyle.

Triggers and Solutions Emotional eating can feel like an insurmountable obstacle on the path to sustainable weight loss. It's common to turn to food for comfort in times of stress, sadness, or even boredom, and for many, these emotional triggers are deeply ingrained. But recognizing these triggers is the first step toward finding solutions that empower you to break free from the cycle of emotional eating.

One of the most significant triggers of emotional eating is stress. When you're stressed, your body releases cortisol, a hormone that can increase your appetite and lead to a craving for sugary or high-fat foods. These foods temporarily boost your mood but often leave you feeling worse in the long run. Combatting stress-induced eating starts with understanding what stresses you out. Creating a stress diary can be helpful; jot down what you feel when you're eating due to stress and notice patterns. Knowing the cause is half the battle, allowing you to strategize on addressing it effectively.

Try implementing stress-reducing techniques that don't involve food. Activities like yoga, meditation, or a simple walk can be instrumental in lowering stress levels. These activities not only distract from the urge to eat but also contribute to your overall well-being. Moreover, integrating these stress management tools into your routine strengthens your ability to handle stress without turning to the pantry.

Another critical trigger is loneliness or feeling isolated. People often eat to fill a void, mistaking a craving for connection as a craving for food. In these moments, reaching out to a friend or joining a group activity can fulfill your need for social interaction, which might be what you're truly craving. Loneliness as a trigger underscores the importance of building a supportive network. Your support system can double as a motivator, encouraging healthier coping strategies that don't involve food.

It's essential to recognize that sometimes, emotional eating stems from unresolved emotions—anger, disappointment, or sadness. Repressing these emotions leads to them manifesting in other areas, such as eating habits. Journaling can be an effective way to process your emotions constructively. This practice allows you to articulate feelings that might otherwise remain bottled up. As you become more attuned to your emotional landscape, you'll likely note a decrease in emotional eating episodes.

Moreover, having a plan for emotional eating is crucial. Consider creating a list of non-food-related activities that can serve as go-to alternatives when you're feeling the urge to eat emotionally. This list could include taking a warm bath, reading a book, or engaging in a creative hobby. By having ready alternatives, you're less likely to default to eating when emotions run high.

The influence of environment as a trigger for emotional eating shouldn't be underestimated. Particularly, the role environmental cues play in prompting us to reach for unhealthy snacks is significant. Placing healthier, more nutritious food options within easy reach can shift the odds in your favor. If you know that you often reach for junk food when watching TV, for example, keep cut-up veggies or nuts handy instead.

Preemptively addressing these environmental triggers can prevent emotional eating before it starts. Rearrange your kitchen to make indulgent snacks less accessible, and remember that out of sight often means out of mind. This conscious adjustment in your environment sets a stage conducive to healthier choices even before an emotional eating trigger arises. Importantly, be kind to yourself throughout this process. Guilt and shame associated with emotional eating can perpetuate the cycle, leaving you caught in a loop. Replace self-criticism with self-compassion, understanding that slip-ups are part of the journey. Viewing these moments as opportunities for growth rather than as failures helps build a more positive mindset around eating.

Finally, if you find that emotional eating remains unmanageable despite your best efforts, seeking professional help can be invaluable. Therapy or counseling can provide specialized strategies tailored to your unique experiences and triggers. These professionals can help structure an environment where emotional eating is no longer the go-to response, guiding you toward healthier, more sustainable coping mechanisms.

While triggers for emotional eating are diverse and personal, solutions exist that align with healthier weight-loss goals. Understanding your emotional landscape and how it connects with your eating habits is empowering. By introducing strategies and solutions that address these emotional triggers, you're nurturing a life where food is no longer a source of comfort but a tool for nourishment and well-being.

Mindful Eating Practices

At its heart, mindful eating isn't about following a strict set of rules or depriving yourself of certain foods. Instead, it's about cultivating a deeper awareness of the eating experience, allowing you to make thoughtful choices that satisfy both your hunger and your mind. We often eat on autopilot, rushing through meals while multitasking, which makes it easy to consume more than we need without truly enjoying what we consume. Breaking free from this cycle requires us to slow down and bring our full attention to the act of eating.

An effective way to start practicing mindful eating is by tuning in to your body's hunger and fullness signals. Before reaching for a snack or sitting down for a meal, pause to ask yourself: "Am I truly hungry?" This simple question can shift your perspective and make you more attuned to the subtle cues your body sends. For many individuals, this alone is a revelation—realizing that emotional triggers, rather than genuine hunger, often prompt them to eat. Acknowledge these emotions without judgment and find alternative ways to address them, such as taking a walk or engaging in a creative hobby.

Moreover, the environment in which you eat plays a crucial role in how you experience food. Set the stage by minimizing distractions like TV or scrolling through your phone, which can detract from the meal's sensory enjoyment. Instead, create a pleasant atmosphere with calming music or a comfortable setting, encouraging you to savor each bite. Notice the colors, textures, and aromas that make up your dish. By focusing on these sensory experiences, you'll not only appreciate your meal more, but also feel more satisfied, which can reduce the urge to overeat.

Another core component of mindful eating is understanding your food's origin and its journey to your plate. Where does it come from? Who prepared it? Contemplate the effort and the process that brought the food to you. This mindful reflection fosters gratitude and a positive connection with your nourishment. You might find yourself naturally drawn to choosing more nutritious and sustainably sourced foods, aligning your choices with your personal values. This alignment isn't just good for your body and mind—it's also kind to the planet.

Developing mindful eating habits takes practice and patience. It's a journey, not a destination, and it's perfectly normal to experience setbacks along the way. Be compassionate with yourself. Mindfulness is a skill that improves over time with consistent practice. Start with one meal a day, dedicating a set amount of time to focus purely on eating mindfully. Gradually, let these practices permeate more of your meals until they become intuitive.

The benefits of mindful eating extend beyond weight loss. By fostering a healthier relationship with food, you can alleviate stress and reduce the guilt often associated with eating. This approach transforms eating from a mundane task into an enriching experience that supports not only physical well-being but also emotional and psychological health. You'll likely discover a newfound freedom in making food choices, guided by genuine self-awareness rather than external pressures or fleeting trends.

Empower yourself with the knowledge that you have the ability to connect deeply with your body's needs. As you embrace mindful eating, you'll find it easier to establish sustainable habits that honor both your health and happiness. You deserve to enjoy your meals, to appreciate every morsel, and to experience the peace that comes with true

Developing Healthy Eating Habits is a journey, not unlike learning a new language. Just as you immerse yourself in conversation to become fluent, you can gradually adopt mindful eating practices to develop a healthier relationship with food. This isn't about deprivation; it's about awareness and choice, and ultimately, it's empowering.

Mindful eating begins with intention—the conscious decision to connect with your body's nutritional needs and emotions surrounding food. It demands you slow down, savor each bite, and focus on the present moment. This practice can transform the way you approach meals, shifting away from automatic, habit-driven consumption to a more thoughtful, deliberate experience. Really, it's less about rigid rules and more about understanding and responding to the signals your body is sending.

Consider this: the simple act of recognizing hunger and satiety cues can be profoundly transformative. Many of us have either ignored or overridden these signals for years, often eating due to boredom, stress, or social situations. By tuning into your body's natural rhythms, you can start to trust your instincts again, eating when you're hungry and stopping when satisfied. As if rediscovering an inner compass, you learn to align your eating with your body's genuine needs.

But let's face it, retraining your brain to eat mindfully takes patience and practice. It is normal to find yourself zoning out during meals, especially in today's fast-paced world. One effective tool here is to eliminate distractions while eating. Try to avoid eating in front of screens or devices. Instead, commit to sitting down at a table, where you can fully engage with your meal, noticing textures and flavors with each bite.

Adopting mindful eating habits also involves questioning lifelong beliefs about food. Consider the role of cultural and familial influences on your eating patterns; these can run deep and often without your conscious awareness. Reflect on how these have shaped your perception of food, and use this awareness to challenge food-related assumptions that no longer serve you. Opening your mind in this way leads to greater food freedom and emotional well-being.

Variety, too, plays a crucial role. Make it your mission to explore a diverse range of foods, enjoying and appreciating each for its unique nutritional profile. Cultivating curiosity about what you put on your plate not only keeps meals exciting but can also improve your nutritional balance over time. Imagine the vibrant colors of fresh produce or the richness of whole grains as allies in your journey—not just staples on your grocery list.

Equally important is honoring your cravings without judgment, seeing them as signals rather than signs of weakness. Acknowledging your desire for certain flavors—whether sweet, salty, or savory—offers insights into your body's needs at any given time. With mindful intention, you can indulge thoughtfully, in moderation, and without guilt, letting go of restrictive mentalities that create unnecessary stress and tension.

For many, setting small, achievable goals provides a helpful framework as they transition to new eating practices. Perhaps you start by introducing one new mindful habit each week, like sitting down to eat or taking five deep breaths before each meal. These manageable steps can gradually lead to more profound changes, reinforcing a sense of accomplishment along the way. Unlike lofty and often unsustainable resolutions, these incremental changes build confidence and ensure consistency.

Community support can be incredibly beneficial as well. Engaging with others who are also seeking to embrace mindful eating creates a supportive environment that encourages nourishment. Mindful eating offers a path to not only achieve weight management goals but also, more importantly, to cultivate a balanced, fulfilled life.

Chapter 5: Psychology of Eating

Understanding the psychology of eating can be transformative for those aiming to lose weight sustainably. Eating isn't just a physical act; it's deeply intertwined with our emotions, memories, and habits. Often, when we reach for food, we're not satisfying hunger, but rather a need for comfort, stress relief, or even boredom. Recognizing this behavior is the first step toward change.

Emotional eating is a common hurdle. We've all experienced moments when stress, sadness, or even joy has led us to consume more than we intended. This isn't about lack of willpower; it's about coping mechanisms. Identifying your triggers—those moments when food becomes a go-to for managing emotions—is crucial. By becoming aware of these moments, you open the door to finding healthier ways to cope. Perhaps a walk, a chat with a friend, or meditation can provide the same relief without the caloric intake.

One effective way to tackle emotional eating is through *mindful eating*. Mindful eating is about being present with your food—truly savoring each bite, noting its texture, flavor, and aroma. This practice encourages you to slow down and recognize your body's hunger and satisfaction signals. Not only can this lead to more enjoyable meals, but it can also prevent overeating by allowing your body time to communicate its needs.

To start practicing mindful eating, one tip is to eliminate distractions during meals. Turn off the TV, put down your phone, and focus on your plate. Engage all your senses by noting the colors, smells, and sounds around you. Take small bites and chew thoroughly, paying attention to how the food tastes and feels in your mouth. Reflect on how you feel before, during, and after your meal to gauge your hunger and satiety levels accurately.

Another tool in understanding the psychology of eating involves self-compassion. It's easy to fall into a cycle of guilt and shame when you indulge or overeat. However, these feelings can sabotage long-term success. Instead, approach these moments with kindness and learning in mind. Why did it happen? What can you do differently next time? Treat yourself with the same empathy you would a friend in a similar situation.

Finally, it's essential to remember that changing your eating habits is a personal journey. There's no one-size-fits-all solution, and what works for someone else might not work for you. Reflect on your unique relationship with food and be honest with yourself about how it's impacting your life. By gaining insights into your eating patterns and empowering yourself with strategies like mindful eating, you set the foundation for a healthier, more balanced approach to both food and weight management. This psychological shift is as vital as the physical changes you're aiming to achieve.

enhancement. Instead of seeing them as opposing forces, imagine them as complementary partners in a balanced fitness plan.

Strength training might challenge you to step beyond your comfort zone, but the rewards are worth the effort. Imagine not only reaching your weight loss goals but also maintaining them with strength and vitality. It's a transformation that's more than skin-deep, influencing your entire lifestyle and outlook on health.

Empowerment comes from understanding the profound impact strength training has on your metabolism and weight loss journey. By building muscle, you're not just shaping a body; you're fostering a life of health and sustainability. With each rep and each set, you're investing in a future free from the yo-yo dieting cycle, underpinned by the power of a revved-up metabolism and a robust physical frame.

As we conclude this section, remember that muscles aren't just for athletes or gym enthusiasts. They're for anyone committed to enriching their lives with energy and health. Incorporate strength training into your regime, complement it with a balanced diet, and witness a transformative change. In the grand scheme of weight loss, muscle is your steadfast ally, ever ready to power your journey towards lasting success.

accountability. This network can either be formal, such as a group program, or informal, like a buddy system. Sharing experiences and challenges with others makes the journey less isolating and much more enriching.

Over time, cultivating these habits shapes how you perceive yourself and your relationship with food. Eating becomes an act of self-care, a chance to nourish your body and soul. This shift not only aids in weight management but also enhances your quality of life, fostering feelings of gratitude and contentment.

In essence, developing healthy eating habits through mindful practice reconnects you to the innate wisdom of your body. It sets the stage for sustainable weight loss by encouraging balance and moderation in ways that rigid dieting never can. While it may require effort and experimentation, the rewards—both physical and emotional—are well worth it. And remember, it's a lifelong practice, not a destination. As you embark on this path, embrace each small victory, knowing they pave the way for enduring change.

Chapter 6: Importance of Sleep in Weight Loss

Weight loss often brings to mind images of restrictive diets, intense workouts, and relentless discipline. Yet, one crucial element frequently slips under the radar: sleep. In the quest for a healthier body, many people overlook the power of a good night's rest. Sleep is not merely a passive state where the body shuts down; it's an active and complex process vital to our overall health, including weight management. Understanding this connection between sleep and weight loss could be the missing piece in your journey to a healthier, more balanced lifestyle.

During sleep, your body performs an orchestra of intricate processes that are essential for both physical and mental health. For starters, sleep affects the hormones that regulate hunger and appetite—specifically, leptin and ghrelin. These are like the body's hunger on-off switches. Leptin signals fullness to your brain, while ghrelin tells you when it's time to eat. Lack of sleep throws this balance out of whack. Studies show that when we don't get enough sleep, ghrelin levels rise and leptin levels drop, which results in increased hunger and appetite.

Moreover, chronic sleep deprivation can lead to insulin resistance, a condition where the body's cells become less responsive to insulin. Insulin is the hormone responsible for helping cells absorb glucose for energy. When cells resist insulin, glucose stays in the bloodstream, leading to high blood sugar levels, which can eventually trigger weight gain and increase the risk of developing type 2 diabetes. This chain reaction underscores why adequate sleep should feature prominently in any weight loss plan.

It's not just about quantity, though. Sleep quality matters just as much. Poor sleep, characterized by frequent awakenings or difficulty falling back asleep, can similarly disrupt hormonal balance and metabolic function. Striving for deep, restful sleep allows the body to fully engage in vital processes that support metabolic health. Prioritizing activities that promote good sleep hygiene—such as establishing a regular sleep schedule, creating a relaxing bedtime routine, and avoiding screens before bed—can make a significant difference in sleep quality.

So, how can good sleep possibly inspire weight loss? Think of sleep as the recharging period for your entire system. When well-rested, you wake up refreshed and ready to tackle the physical and mental challenges of the day, including those related to weight loss. With your energy reserves full, you're more likely to stick to workout plans and make nutritious food choices. Adequate sleep enhances mood and focus, reducing the likelihood of stress eating or succumbing to junk food cravings.

This isn't just theory; research backs up these claims. Studies indicate that individuals who consistently sleep less than seven hours a night are more likely to have higher body mass indexes (BMIs) than those who sleep a healthy amount. A well-rested individual commands strong decision-making abilities, a crucial asset when making lifestyle changes for the better.

Achieving a healthy weight is an integration of sustaining small yet meaningful habits over time. Incorporating sleep as a non-negotiable component of your routine will not only benefit your waistline but elevate your overall well-being. It's about recognizing that alongside diet and exercise, sleep is the third pillar that supports your health goals. Thus, by ensuring you give yourself the luxury of rest, you set the stage for long-term success in your weight loss journey. You empower yourself to face the challenges ahead with vigor, clarity, and resilience.

In the end, embracing the importance of sleep means acknowledging its rightful place in the tapestry of your life and weight loss efforts. You're not just aiming for a number on a scale but a holistic sense of health. Let sleep be the unsung hero in your journey to weight loss; you'll find that it rewards you tenfold with its transformative power.

How Sleep Affects Hormones

It's remarkable how intertwined sleep and hormones are in the body's quest for balance, especially in relation to weight management. When you don't get enough quality sleep, a cascade of hormonal shifts occurs that can significantly impact your weight loss efforts. Hormones like cortisol, insulin, ghrelin, and leptin are key players in this area, and understanding their roles can be a game changer on your journey to sustainable weight loss.

Let's start with cortisol, often dubbed 'the stress hormone.' When you skimp on sleep, your body perceives stress, and cortisol levels spike to help you stay alert. Unfortunately, this can increase your appetite, leading you to consume more calories, particularly in the form of carbs and sugars. Over time, elevated cortisol levels can contribute to weight gain, especially around the abdomen, making it a formidable adversary in weight management. Insulin, another critical hormone, is responsible for managing your blood sugar levels. Poor sleep can cause insulin sensitivity to decrease, making it harder for your body to process glucose efficiently. This can lead to higher blood sugar levels and, ultimately, increase the risk of storing more body fat. The interplay between insulin and sleep highlights the importance of regular sleep patterns for maintaining a healthy weight.

Two other hormonal players, ghrelin and leptin, often called the "hunger hormones," are directly affected by sleep. Ghrelin tells your brain when to eat, while leptin signals when you're full. Lack of sleep increases ghrelin levels—causing you to crave more food—and decreases leptin levels, making you feel less satisfied after eating. This double whammy can result in overeating and weight gain.

Additionally, sleep influences growth hormone production, which plays a role in muscle repair and growth as well as fat burning. During deep sleep, your body releases growth hormones, promoting muscle recovery and growth that aid in metabolism boosting. A lack of deep sleep interrupts this process, making it harder to lose weight and maintain muscle mass.

On a more positive note, prioritizing sleep can naturally correct these hormonal imbalances, setting a stable foundation for weight loss. Simple adjustments such as creating a bedtime routine, reducing screen time before bed, and managing stress can promote better sleep quality and duration. These practices not only help regulate hormone levels but also enhance overall well-being, fostering a more balanced approach to weight loss. Ultimately, acknowledging and addressing the role of sleep in regulating hormones could be one of the most effective, yet often overlooked strategies in your weight loss toolbox. It's a natural, foundational element that supports not just your weight goals, but your health as a whole, reinforcing the fact that meaningful lifestyle changes are never solely about diet or exercise alone. By understanding the crucial connection between sleep and hormones, you empower yourself to make informed choices that support both your health and weight loss journey.

The Link Between Sleep Quality and Weight delves into one of the most underappreciated aspects of weight management. It's easy to underestimate the impact of restful sleep on our health, especially in a culture that often prizes productivity over well-being. Yet, when we consider how sleep affects our hormones, we begin to see why quality sleep is essential for those striving for effective and sustainable weight loss.

Stillness in the night signals to the body that it's time to balance critical hormones like cortisol, ghrelin, and leptin. These are the chemical messengers that help regulate appetite, stress, and energy storage, respectively. Missing out on quality sleep can throw these hormonal balances off kilter, driving us toward habits that hinder weight loss. When you don't sleep well, your body produces more ghrelin, the hormone that signals hunger, and less leptin, the one that tells you when you're full. This imbalance can lead to a greater appetite and increased caloric intake.

Research consistently illustrates how inadequate sleep contributes to weight gain. A study involving more than 1,000 participants found that those sleeping fewer than six hours per night had a significantly higher risk of becoming overweight compared to those enjoying more than seven hours of rest. There's a reason for this—that deficit of just a couple of hours changes the hormonal milieu, favoring hunger and food cravings.

On top of that, cortisol levels spike when you're sleep-deprived. Cortisol is the stress hormone that tells your body to conserve energy, a survival mechanism that makes your body hold onto fat stores—especially around your midsection. Over time, chronically high cortisol levels lead not only to weight gain but also to difficulties in losing those extra pounds. Stressful days lead into sleepless nights, creating a vicious cycle of weight struggles that can feel difficult to break.

But don't despair. Understanding the connection between sleep quality and hormones provides a powerful insight. It can inspire you to prioritize rest as part of your weight loss strategy. Start by establishing a sleep routine that provides calm and consistency. Going to bed and waking up at the same time each day anchors your body's internal clock, making it easier to fall asleep and stay asleep.

Remember, your sleep environment needs to be conducive to rest. Keep your bedroom cool, dark, and quiet. Try to disconnect from screens at least an hour before bedtime, as the blue light emitted by phones, tablets, and computers can trick your brain into thinking it's still daytime, making it harder to wind down. Engaging in a relaxing activity, whether it's reading a book or practicing meditation, can also set the tone for slumber.

Moreover, consider how your diet influences sleep quality. Consuming heavy meals or caffeine too close to bedtime can disrupt your sleep, according to numerous studies. Similarly, eating a balanced diet with sufficient nutrients can promote better rest, indirectly supporting your weight loss efforts. Foods rich in magnesium, such as leafy greens, and those containing tryptophan, like turkey and bananas, can help in this regard.

An often overlooked component of sleep is its role in recovery from physical activity, which is another key pillar of weight loss. During deep sleep, the body repairs muscles, strengthens bones, and rejuvenates tissues—all crucial processes after a day of workouts. Thus, without enough rest, not only does hormonal imbalance make weight loss more challenging, but physical recovery is compromised as well.

In sum, the art of weight loss is not solely about eating less or moving more. It's about creating a harmonious balance between all aspects of your life—diet, exercise, and most definitely, sleep. Recognize the vital role sleep plays, not as a passive rest period but as a powerful tool in your weight loss arsenal. Aiming for those seven to nine hours of sleep could be as important as any diet or exercise regimen you choose to follow.

As you integrate this knowledge into your life, you'll discover that prioritizing quality sleep not only transforms your weight loss journey but enriches your overall health and well-being. Let the power of good sleep guide you toward your goals, offering you the energy, clarity, and balance you need to succeed in sustainable weight loss. With patience and persistence, allow sleep to be the steady rhythm that drives your progress and supports your transformation.

Chapter 7: Managing Stress for Effective Weight Loss

In the quest for effective and sustainable weight loss, managing stress emerges as a pivotal element often overlooked. Stress, as a silent architect, shapes our habits, choices, and ultimately, our waistlines. For many, the journey towards shedding pounds is fraught with tension and anxiety, often making it harder to adhere to a routine that's both healthful and consistent. The relationship between stress and weight is a complex dance, influencing both physiological and behavioral patterns that can hinder your weight loss efforts if left unchecked.

It's crucial to understand how stress impacts your body and why it can be a formidable barrier to weight loss. When you're stressed, your body releases cortisol, a hormone that, among other things, can lead to increased appetite and cravings for sugary or fatty foods. These high-caloric desires have little to do with your actual nutritional needs and more to do with your body's response to surviving what it perceives as a threat. Over time, elevated cortisol levels are linked to weight gain, particularly around the abdomen, which poses increased health risks.

But the effects of stress aren't just physiological; they seep into every decision we make. Stress can drive us towards emotional eating, where food becomes a source of comfort rather than nourishment. This habit often leads to overconsumption and disruptions in achieving nutritional balance. Furthermore, stress can sap the motivation needed to exercise, meditate, or engage in activities that foster a healthy lifestyle. All these contribute to a potentially vicious cycle where stress creates weight gain, and weight gain, in turn, creates more stress.

Breaking this cycle begins with acknowledging stress as a tangible, manageable challenge in your weight loss journey. Taking proactive steps to reduce stress can dramatically enhance your capacity for effective weight management. Techniques such as mindfulness meditation, regular physical activity, and adequate sleep can significantly lower stress levels. Simple practices like deep breathing or setting aside just ten minutes a day for relaxation can have an outsized impact, bringing both tranquility and renewed energy. Mindfulness, specifically, helps ground you in the present moment, reducing the overwhelming nature of stress. By practicing mindfulness, you reconnect with the sensations of your body and the emotions you feel, without judgment. This awareness encourages more intentional choices, be it in the food you eat or the extent of your daily physical activity. Similarly, integrating physical exercise is not just about burning calories but also about boosting endorphins, the body's natural stress relievers.

Building resilience against stress also involves creating an environment that supports calmness and well-being. Consider structuring your surroundings to reduce common stress triggers. This might mean organizing your home to promote a sense of peace, perhaps by decluttering or adding elements like plants and relaxing music that enhance calm. Additionally, maintaining a supportive social network can play a vital role in stress management. Sharing experiences and challenges with friends or family often helps reduce stress and improves your motivation and accountability.

Another crucial aspect of stress management is ensuring you get enough sleep. Quality sleep is a robust protector against stress. During sleep, your body undergoes processes vital for managing stress levels, like reducing cortisol production and repairing tissues. Consistently sleeping fewer hours than needed not only heightens stress levels but also affects the hormones governing hunger, contributing to increased appetite and cravings. Prioritizing a consistent sleep schedule can therefore be one of the most straightforward yet impactful strategies to combat weight gain associated with stress.

Ultimately, harnessing the power of stress management for weight loss is about integration and consistency. It's not solely about de-stressing once or twice when you feel overwhelmed. Instead, it's about adopting lifestyle changes that make effective coping mechanisms second nature. These include regularly scheduled personal time, maintaining hobbies that cultivate joy, and navigating challenges with a mindset geared toward growth and learning. This approach fosters a resilient, empowered mindset—vital in the ongoing path of weight loss and overall well-being.

In managing stress thoughtfully and proactively, you not only unlock pathways towards effective weight loss but also enhance the quality of your life in ways beyond the scale. As you incorporate stress reduction strategies into your daily routine, remember that patience and persistence are key. The gentle, persistent removal of mental weight often lightens physical weight recalcitrant to any diet or exercise plan. In understanding stress's profound influence on your body and behavior, you gain a powerful tool, not just for losing weight, but for living a fuller, more vibrant life.

Stress and Its Impact on Body Weight

In the pursuit of effective weight loss, stress often emerges as a formidable adversary. It's a common, yet overlooked factor that could dramatically affect one's body weight. When the pressures of life mount, whether from work, relationships, or finances, our bodies react in ways that can sabotage our best efforts to lose weight. Understanding how stress affects body weight is crucial for anyone on a journey toward sustainable weight loss.

When we're stressed, our bodies release hormones like cortisol and adrenaline, preparing us for a fight-or-flight response. This primitive reaction, useful in the early days of human evolution to escape predators, isn't quite suitable for modern-day stressors like deadlines or arguments. Elevated cortisol levels, in particular, can lead to increased appetite, encouraging us to reach for comfort foods high in sugar and fat. These are the types of foods that can quickly derail our weight loss goals.

Moreover, stress affects our bodies on a cellular level. It can alter our metabolism, making it harder to shed pounds even when sticking to a strict diet and exercise regime. Stress can also lead to sleep disturbances, which further disrupts hormonal balance, including hormones that regulate hunger and satiety. This cycle of stress, poor sleep, and hormonal imbalance sets the stage for potential weight gain, creating a frustrating loop for those trying to lose weight.

It's not just the biological mechanisms of stress that affect body weight. Behavioral changes in response to stress play a significant role as well. Many people tend to eat emotionally when stressed, seeking solace in food as a way to cope with their feelings. This pattern, known as emotional eating, can lead to the consumption of excess calories and make weight control even more challenging. Identifying and managing emotional triggers is essential to breaking this cycle.

There's also a social aspect to stress and how it affects weight. When people are stressed, they might skip workouts or avoid physical activity altogether due to feeling overwhelmed or too tired. Social support systems can become strained, leading to isolation or reduced motivation to engage in healthy behaviors. In the absence of supportive friends or family, individuals might resort to unhealthy habits that counteract their weight loss efforts.

Fortunately, understanding stress's impact on body weight opens the door to targeted interventions and strategies to mitigate its effects. Mind-body practices like yoga and meditation have shown promise in reducing stress levels, helping individuals regain control over their physiological responses. By practicing mindfulness, we can become more aware of our body's cues and prevent stress from dictating our eating behaviors.

Engaging in regular physical activity is another powerful antidote to stress. Exercise acts as a stress reliever by promoting the production of endorphins, which are natural mood lifters. Incorporating activities that are enjoyable and fulfilling, rather than seen as a chore, can increase adherence to an exercise regimen and gradually reduce stress levels over time.

Additionally, setting realistic expectations and goals in the weight loss journey can alleviate some of the stress that comes from feeling pressured to achieve rapid results. Celebrating small milestones, rather than focusing entirely on the end goal, can keep motivation high and stress levels low. Building a balanced lifestyle that respects personal limits and prioritizes mental health is essential.

Incorporating stress management techniques into a weight loss plan is not an indulgence but a necessary component of achieving lasting results. By addressing the root of stress and its manifestations, individuals can create a healthier relationship with food and exercise, fostering an environment where sustainable weight loss is possible.

Ultimately, tackling stress's impact on body weight requires a holistic approach that acknowledges both the physical and mental dimensions of health. Understanding the profound connection between stress and weight empowers individuals to make informed choices that benefit not only their waistlines but also their overall well-being. Remember, the path to effective weight loss is just as much about managing life's stresses as it is about diet and exercise.

Techniques to Reduce Stress-related Weight Gain take center stage in our journey toward effective weight management. Stress, undoubtedly, affects many aspects of our lives, including body weight. When life feels overwhelming, it's common to turn to food for comfort, which might lead to unwelcome weight gain. Fortunately, there are strategies you can employ to reduce the impact of stress on your weight.

First off, acknowledging the relationship between stress and weight gain is crucial. When you experience stress, your body releases cortisol, a hormone that can increase appetite and lead to cravings, particularly for high-sugar or high-fat foods. This biological response is a survival mechanism dating back to our ancestors who needed extra energy in times of danger. In today's world, though, this can translate into unwanted pounds.

One of the most effective techniques is *mindful eating*. It's not just about what you eat, but how you eat. When stressed, we tend to eat quickly and without thought. Mindful eating encourages you to slow down and savor each bite, paying attention to your hunger and fullness cues. It's about making a conscious effort to enjoy your food and recognize when you've had enough. This practice helps you develop a healthier relationship with food and can reduce stress-related eating.

Incorporating relaxation techniques into your daily routine can also mitigate stress. Practices such as meditation, deep breathing exercises, and yoga are excellent ways to calm the mind, decrease cortisol levels, and promote a sense of balance. Meditation, for instance, encourages a focus on the present moment, which can alleviate stress by reducing worries about the past and future. Similarly, yoga combines physical movement with mindful breathing, creating a synergy that enhances both physical and mental well-being.

Moreover, getting active in ways that you enjoy can be a natural stress-buster. Regular physical activity doesn't just help burn calories; it boosts endorphins, which elevate mood and alleviate stress. Find activities that you genuinely enjoy, whether it's hiking, cycling, dancing, or simply taking a walk in the park. When exercise is enjoyable, you'll be more likely to stick with it, creating a positive feedback loop that benefits both your mental health and waistline.

Another practical approach is ensuring a good night's sleep, as poor sleep can exacerbate stress and disrupt hunger-regulating hormones. Create a nighttime routine that includes winding down from technology and setting a regular sleep schedule. Your body needs rest to recover, and quality sleep can help manage both stress levels and weight.

Lastly, don't underestimate the power of social connections. Sharing your journey with friends or joining a support group can significantly reduce stress. Conversations and interactions with others can provide comfort, encouragement, and a feeling of belonging, which can buffer against stress and related weight gain.

Incorporating these techniques into your lifestyle requires intention and practice. By adopting mindful eating, relaxation practices, regular exercise, prioritizing sleep, and seeking support, you can effectively manage stress and prevent it from sabotaging your weight loss efforts. Remember, in the quest for lasting weight loss, understanding and managing the influence of stress is just as important as dietary and exercise changes.

Chapter 8: Building a Support System

Embarking on a weight loss journey is a commendable decision, but it can sometimes feel daunting and isolating. That's why constructing a robust support system is not just beneficial—it's essential. Just like any meaningful transformation, achieving sustainable weight loss isn't solely about personal willpower or dietary choices. It's also about surrounding yourself with people who uplift you, share in your successes, and offer a hand during setbacks.

The role of social support in weight loss is profound. Studies have shown that people who forge supportive networks are more likely to achieve their weight loss goals compared to those who go it alone. Friends and family aren't just bystanders; they become your cheerleaders and sometimes even your workout partners. They help keep you accountable, celebrate your milestones, and most importantly, remind you of your 'why' when times get tough.

However, while having a network of friends and family is invaluable, it's also wise to seek professional guidance. Nutritionists and personal trainers can provide tailored advice and objective insights that your loved ones might not be equipped to offer. These professionals have the expertise to devise personalized plans that consider your unique needs and circumstances.

A nutritionist can help you navigate the often confusing landscape of dietary needs and preferences; they offer clarity and direction where confusion might otherwise reign. Similarly, a personal trainer can teach you how to exercise effectively, ensuring that you're getting the most out of your workouts. They can guide you through various exercises, ensuring proper form and emphasizing activities that complement your weight loss objectives.

Your support system doesn't have to be just physical. In today's digital age, virtual communities can offer a plethora of support options. Online forums, social media groups, and wellness apps often host communities where you can share experiences, exchange tips, and find motivation from like-minded individuals all over the world. The key is to find a community that aligns with your values and goals, one that feels like a natural extension of your support system.

Building a support system is, in itself, an act of empowerment. It signifies the understanding that while your journey is personal, you don't have to walk it alone. Every relationship you nurture and professional you consult contributes another brick to a foundation that supports your long-term health. Never underestimate the power of a kind word or the motivational push a good support system can provide.

In the end, the journey to lasting weight loss is as much about connection as it is about calorie counting and exercise routines. So, reach out and build your support system with intention and care—it'll make all the difference in your pursuit of health and happiness.

The Role of Social Support in Weight Loss

Embarking on a weight loss journey can feel overwhelming, but having a solid support system can make all the difference. When it comes to achieving sustainable weight loss, the encouragement and accountability that comes from social support is invaluable. Whether it's from family, friends, or a weight loss community, social support reinforces commitment, provides motivation, and creates a sense of belonging that can propel you toward your goals.

The power of social support lies in its ability to foster accountability. When you share your goals with others, you're making a commitment not just to yourself, but also to them. This can be incredibly motivating, as the expectation of others can push you to stay on track, even when you're tempted to stray. It's not just about accountability, though—connection is also key. In a world that can sometimes feel isolating, having people who understand your struggles and cheer you on can reduce feelings of isolation and boost your morale. It's comforting to know you're walking this path with others who are invested in your success.

Beyond accountability, social support provides emotional sustenance along the journey. Weight loss can evoke a whirlwind of emotions—from frustration during plateaus to exhilaration with progress. Having a network that offers empathy and encouragement during the tough times and celebrates victories, no matter how small, can enhance your resilience. It's about cultivating a space where emotions are validated, and struggles are acknowledged. With support, you're more likely to persevere through challenges, knowing there's a safety net ready to catch you.

Moreover, the collective wisdom of a support group can't be underestimated. When it comes to practical advice, from meal prep tips to workout ideas, crowd-sourcing knowledge can open doors to new strategies you might not have considered. Supportive communities are often treasure troves of information, offering innovative solutions that resonate because they've been tried and tested by others facing the same hurdles. This shared learning experience can spark creativity and provide a fresh perspective on overcoming obstacles.

Incorporating social support into your weight loss approach doesn't mean that you have to open your life to scrutiny. It can be as simple as finding a buddy for regular walks or joining an online group where members share similar goals. The key is to find environments that are positive and nurturing, avoiding spaces that breed negativity or competition. Not all support is created equal, and it's crucial to surround yourself with individuals who lift you up, not bring you down.

Finally, remember that building a support network is a two-way street. Being a source of support for others not only enriches your journey but also reinforces your commitment to your own goals. Encouragement and empathy you offer can feel just as rewarding as what you receive, creating a cycle of support that perpetuates positivity and success. Embracing social support as part of your weight loss strategy transforms what could be a solitary challenge into a shared adventure, where strength is found in numbers and success is celebrated together.

How Friends and Family Can Help Leaning on friends and family during your weight loss journey can make a significant difference. While you're the one making choices about what to eat and how to move your body, having a network of support amplifies your efforts. The people closest to you can serve as motivators, cheerleaders, and even accountability partners. They've got the potential to help you stay on track and make sure your healthy habits stick. But how they can help and all the little ways they can encourage you requires some understanding and communication.

First and foremost, it's crucial to communicate your goals and needs to those around you. Maybe you're swapping late-night snacks for a cup of herbal tea, or you've decided to wake up an hour early to fit in a morning jog. Whatever it is, share these changes with your friends and family. When they know what you're aiming for, they can much more effectively offer support and encouragement. And don't worry—sharing doesn't mean you're burdening them. In fact, people generally feel honored to be included in your journey and happy to help you flourish. It's about creating an environment that fosters your growth and relieves some of the pressure you might be feeling.

Moreover, having someone to talk to when challenges arise adds a layer of protection against reverting to old habits. Suppose you're feeling discouraged after a week without visible progress; a supportive friend or family member can remind you of how far you've come and why you shouldn't give up. Emotional support acts as a glue holding together the various pieces of your weight loss strategy. Conversations don't need to be all about weight and food; sometimes, the best support is a distraction—a good laugh or a shared activity that takes your mind off the struggle.

Incorporating those you trust into your new routine can make for a more enjoyable experience. Rather than looking at exercise as a solitary endeavor, involve your friends and family. A Saturday hike or an evening walk with a friend turns movement into quality time, allowing you to bond while simultaneously working towards your health goals. Workout buddies offer subtle peer pressure; if they're counting on you to show up, skipping isn't an option without letting someone down.

Then there's the accountability factor. Family and friends can call you out—kindly, of course—when you're veering off track. Maybe you're tempted by an extra slice of cake. A gentle nudge from a loved one can be the reminder you need to stick to your plan. But remember, accountability goes both ways. Make sure you're setting clear rules and boundaries. If you don't want them policing your every move or meal choice, let them know when and how you'd appreciate their involvement. Constructive dialogue around this can prevent resentment and strengthens your relationships.

Celebrating victories, big or small, is another area where friends and family shine. Losing a pound, hitting a milestone, or even just making it through a tough week can feel monumental when acknowledged by others. Their enthusiasm and recognition reinforce your own sense of accomplishment, driving you to maintain the momentum. A shared celebration doesn't just boost your mood, it fortifies your commitment—making you feel that your journey is a shared success.

But it's not only about receiving support; actively involving friends and family in healthier lifestyle choices can be a boon for them too. Encourage them to join in meal prepping or to try out a new healthy recipe with you. Such collective activities promote a supportive environment and might even inspire lifestyle changes in them. By naturally integrating them into your journey, you grow their understanding of your challenges and provide them with knowledge and motivation to alter their habits as well.

There are certainly pitfalls to watch for. Sometimes loved ones, despite their best intentions, can become obstacles. They might unknowingly sabotage your efforts by offering tempting treats or not respecting the limits you've set. This is where having honest but gentle conversations comes in. Discussion builds understanding, and understanding fosters cooperation. By laying everything out in an open and constructive discussion, obstacles can become opportunities for growth in your relationship.

Finally, understand that everyone won't be on board. You may find some loved ones have no interest in changing the status quo. That's perfectly fine too. The key is to focus on those who are willing to support your journey without being distracted by those who aren't. Consistency and open communication will gradually win even the most hesitant family members to at least respect your new path.

In summary, surrounding yourself with friends and family creates a cushion—absorbing stressors and external pressures—leaving you to focus on your journey, lighter and more encouraged. Ensure transparency, engage them in your process, and invite their participation, but do so on your terms. With these foundations, your support system can contribute significantly to your weight loss success, providing not only practical assistance but also emotional reinforcement.

Finding Professional Guidance
Navigating the maze of weight loss can feel overwhelming, but you don't have to tackle it alone. Seeking professional guidance is a valuable step on your journey—one that can provide clarity, expertise, and motivation. Nutritionists and personal trainers are two types of professionals who offer tailored insights that resonate with your personal needs and lifestyle. By tapping into their knowledge, you not only gain specific strategies aligned with scientific principles, but also benefit from their experience in steering away from pitfalls like fad diets or exercise burnout.

Consider working with a nutritionist, who can help you understand the complexities of food as fuel. They offer personalized eating plans that enhance your metabolism and cater to your individual tastes and preferences. More importantly, they demystify common nutritional misconceptions that often derail progress. With a nutritionist's guidance, you're equipped to make informed choices that promote sustainable weight loss, crafted around nutritious, enjoyable meals. Having someone to analyze your current habits and suggest practical, incremental changes transforms the abstract idea of "eating healthy" into achievable, daily actions.

Similarly, engaging with a personal trainer can elevate your fitness journey, turning exercise from a chore into a rewarding routine. Trainers not only design workout protocols that fit your level of experience and goals but also teach you to perform exercises safely and effectively. Their encouragement can push you past mental barriers and into new territories of physical capability, helping you discover the strength you never knew you had. This personalized attention ensures that your exercise routine remains dynamic and adaptable to your evolving needs.

Building a support system with professionals isn't just about receiving instruction—it's also about creating accountability and gaining empowerment. The relationships you forge with such experts tailor a framework for success that is uniquely yours, and this personalized approach is often the missing link in achieving lasting weight loss.

The Benefits of Working with Nutritionists and Trainers can be transformative on your weight loss journey, providing guidance and support throughout your quest for a healthier lifestyle. Picture this: a duo of experts dedicated to helping you understand and optimize your unique nutritional and fitness needs. Their collective expertise provides a roadmap that can lead to sustainable and effective weight loss.

Nutritionists bring a wealth of knowledge about food, but they also delve deeper into how nutrition affects every facet of your well-being. They don't just hand you a diet; they educate you about the "why" and "how" of eating. For people tired of fads and misinformation, their insights are not only enlightening but liberating. By analyzing your current eating habits and health goals, nutritionists can provide personalized advice that aligns with your lifestyle, whether you're juggling a busy schedule or managing specific health conditions like diabetes or hypertension.

Equally important is the role of trainers, who specialize in physical activity and exercise programs tailored to your individual needs. Trainers motivate you to push past self-imposed limits, cultivating both strength and confidence. They create diverse exercise routines that prevent monotony and help you discover the joy in movement. Moreover, having a trainer ensures that your workout techniques remain safe and effective, minimizing the risk of injury while maximizing the benefits of your workouts.

One of the greatest advantages of working with both professionals is the collaborative support they offer. Together, nutritionists and trainers can create a comprehensive wellness plan that encompasses both diet and exercise, ensuring that both elements work synergistically. This collaboration can lead to more balanced and sustainable results. When nutritionists and trainers are in sync, the common ground they find is your success.

Another benefit of professional guidance is accountability. Nutritionists and trainers provide the structured support system necessary to keep you on track. They hold you accountable, not in a punitive way, but as partners in your journey. With regular check-ins and progress updates, it's easier to stay motivated. Accountability creates an external expectation to succeed, which can be especially powerful when internal motivation wanes. Moreover, working with professionals allows you to address the psychological aspects of weight loss. Nutritionists often have experience in dealing with emotional eating, helping you uncover triggers and develop coping strategies. Trainers, meanwhile, can help build a positive body image and boost self-esteem through physical accomplishments. This emotional and mental support is crucial in breaking the cycle of negative thinking and cultivating a positive mindset towards weight loss.

For individuals with previous injuries or complex nutritional needs, professionals provide tailored advice that suits these special circumstances. Nutritionists can help incorporate anti-inflammatory foods into your diet while accommodating allergies or intolerances. Trainers can adapt exercises to accommodate or rehabilitate past injuries, ensuring that you still gain strength and vitality without risking further harm. This level of customization is where the true value of professional guidance really shines through.

Communication is another pillar of success when working with nutritionists and trainers. They foster an environment where questions are encouraged, providing explanations that make their strategies relatable and understandable. This transparency ensures that you're not just following instructions but actually learning and adopting new habits to last a lifetime. By forging a relationship built on trust and communication, you are empowered to make informed decisions about your health and well-being.

Lastly, nutritionists and trainers provide a network of support that goes beyond their one-on-one guidance. They often connect you to a community of like-minded individuals, all striving for health and wellness. This community becomes a source of inspiration, sharing stories and tips while cheering each other on. With two experts and a supportive community, your weight loss journey transforms from a solitary challenge into a shared endeavor filled with camaraderie.

In summary, the benefits of working with nutritionists and trainers can't be overstated. They provide professional expertise, personal motivation, tailored plans, accountability, and emotional support. This combination not only enhances your chances of achieving and maintaining weight loss but also redefines how you see health and wellness. Engaging with these professionals sets you on a path where your health goals are not just attainable but enjoyable and sustainable, leading to a richer quality of life.

Chapter 9: Tracking Progress Effectively

As you embark on your weight loss journey, tracking your progress isn't just helpful; it's essential. It's like having a roadmap while traveling across unknown terrain: it tells you where you started, where you are, and where you're headed. Without it, you might find yourself circling back to old habits or feeling lost without tangible evidence of how far you've really come. The habit of consistently and effectively tracking progress can be a beacon of motivation, shining light on accomplishments while illuminating areas that need adjustment.

Choosing the right tools is crucial when you're monitoring your weight loss. Today, we're blessed with a multitude of apps and gadgets that can make tracking more accurate and less intrusive. From smartphone apps that log caloric intake and activity levels to wearable fitness trackers that count steps and measure heart rates, technology offers us a suite of options to keep tabs on our progress. Still, it's important to pick tools that fit seamlessly into your lifestyle. If an app feels cumbersome or a gadget seems more like a ball and chain, it might not be the best choice. Consider what metrics are most valuable to you and select tools that make these insights easily accessible.

Now, let's talk about goal setting. It's a vital part of tracking your progress effectively. Many people set grandiose weight loss goals, expecting massive changes in a short period. The truth is, realistic and achievable goals serve as powerful motivators. Start by breaking down your ultimate objective into smaller, manageable milestones. This not only prevents overwhelm but also allows for a steady stream of victories that keep morale high. For instance, instead of aiming to lose 50 pounds, focus on losing the first five, then the next. Each small win builds momentum.

Tracking isn't solely about numbers on a scale. While weight is a significant indicator, it doesn't tell the whole story. Body measurements, such as waist circumference or body fat percentage, give a fuller picture of your progress. Additionally, take note of non-physical changes: do you have more energy? Are your clothes fitting better? Is your overall mood improving? These, too, are powerful indicators of positive change. Embrace these metrics as they paint a comprehensive picture of your journey beyond just weight loss.

Finally, it's essential to approach tracking with a mindset of curiosity rather than judgment. This journey shouldn't be about scrutinizing every fluctuation as a failure but understanding it as feedback. If the scale isn't moving as quickly as you'd like, don't fret. Look at it as an opportunity to explore deeper. Are your workouts aligned with your goals? Is stress impacting your eating habits? This non-judgmental reflection helps identify patterns and refine strategies without self-criticism.

Incorporating these tracking methods into your routine will not only enhance your success but will help maintain it in the long run. Remember, the ultimate goal isn't a number—it's a healthier, more vibrant version of yourself. Tracking is simply the practice of honoring your commitment to that version, every step of the way.

Tools for Monitoring Weight Loss

Embarking on a weight loss journey can feel like setting sail on uncharted waters. But with the right tools, you can navigate these waters with confidence and track your progress effectively. In today's digital age, a myriad of tools are at your fingertips to aid in monitoring your weight loss journey, from apps to wearable gadgets, making it easier than ever to keep track of your progress.

One of the most accessible and convenient tools for tracking weight loss is the modern smartphone. There are numerous apps available that cater to different aspects of weight management. These apps often provide features such as calorie counting, meal logging, and exercise tracking. MyFitnessPal and Lose It! are great examples of how technology can be your ally in achieving your weight loss goals. They allow you to track your calorie intake effortlessly, providing insights into your dietary habits.

Wearable fitness trackers have become increasingly popular and are powerful tools for monitoring physical activity and weight loss. Devices like Fitbit, Garmin, or Apple Watch not only track your steps and activity levels but also monitor your heart rate and even your sleep patterns. These gadgets can give you a comprehensive view of your health journey, offering data that can be used to adjust your fitness and health routines effectively. The instant feedback provided by these devices can be incredibly motivating, prompting you to move a little more each day.

For those who prefer a more traditional approach, maintaining a handwritten journal can be just as effective. Writing down your meals, workouts, and thoughts about your progress can build a deeper awareness of your behaviors and patterns. Journaling offers reflection time—something digital tools might not—and allows you to see the big picture over time. Plus, it can be a therapeutic process, helping you stay committed to your goals through mindful practice.

Weight scales, both the conventional and smart versions, provide another layer of monitoring. While a conventional scale gives you a basic weight reading, smart scales offer more detailed information such as body fat percentage, muscle mass, and even BMI. These metrics can provide a more well-rounded view of your progress, helping you understand shifts in your body composition that traditional weight readings might miss.

Regardless of the tool you choose, setting realistic and measurable goals is essential. Monitoring tools are most effective when they're used to track progress toward specific, achievable objectives. Regularly reviewing this data can help you stay accountable and adapt your strategies when needed.

Remember, the ultimate aim of using these tools isn't to obsess over numbers but rather to gain insight and awareness about your journey. Whether through technology or more tactile methods, these tools are here to support and empower you in your pursuit of sustainable, healthy weight loss. As you record your victories and learn from setbacks, each entry marks a step forward on your path to a healthier you. With the right tools at your side, you have everything you need to not only track your progress but to celebrate it.

Apps and Gadgets to Track Success play a crucial role in the weight loss journey, providing both tangible metrics and a source of motivation. Imagine having a personal assistant in your pocket—one that not only tracks your every step but also helps manage your calorie intake, sleep patterns, and even water consumption. In today's tech-savvy world, digital tools are indispensable for those looking to shed pounds in a measured and sustainable manner. With a plethora of apps and gadgets available, the challenge often lies in finding the ones that align with your personal goals and lifestyle. These tools offer more than just raw data; they offer insights that can drive long-term change.

The variety in apps and gadgets is vast, catering to different aspects of health and fitness. Activity trackers, such as Fitbit or Garmin, measure steps, heart rate, and even sleep cycles. They're ideal for those who love data-driven insights into their daily activity levels. More comprehensive than a simple pedometer, these devices offer an overview of one's day-to-day physical exertion, allowing for adjustments where needed. Meanwhile, smart scales take the standard bathroom scale to the next level, offering metrics like body fat percentage and muscle mass alongside weight. These additional insights give a fuller picture of one's health, marking progress beyond just a number on the scale.

Among these tools, nutrition tracking apps like MyFitnessPal, Lose It!, or Cronometer deserve a special mention. They help keep tabs on your calorie intake and macronutrient distribution, ensuring you're nourishing your body according to your weight loss plan. The convenience of barcode scanning and large databases makes food entry less of a chore and more of an enlightening meditation on eating habits. This reflection can lead to more informed choices and inevitably, better health outcomes.

What truly sets some of these apps apart is their community features. Platforms like Strava or SparkPeople offer social connectivity that can fuel motivation and accountability. Whether it's sharing your latest run or participating in a group challenge, the sense of camaraderie can be a driving force. Beyond individual tracking, these communities remind us that we're not alone in our journey. They provide a network of support, akin to an online group therapy where shared goals and mutual encouragement thrive.

Progress can also be visualized creatively through apps like Happy Scale or Progress, which focus on trends rather than day-to-day fluctuations. These apps help users celebrate mini milestones and avoid discouragement over minor setbacks. Visualization of progress, be it through graphs or photo journaling, brings a sense of accomplishment that numbers alone may not provide. It emphasizes the journey over the destination, highlighting sustainable changes over quick fixes.

Then, there are gadgets that might seem futuristic yet are becoming more mainstream. Smart drink bottles, for instance, ensure you're staying hydrated with gentle reminders and consumption tracking. Proper hydration is often overlooked in weight loss but is crucial to overall health. Similarly, devices like Lumen claim to offer real-time metabolic data using a simple breath analysis. While these might cater more to biohackers or tech enthusiasts, they represent a growing intersection of health and technology.

However, with all this technology at our fingertips, mindfulness remains an important balance. Gadgets and apps can sometimes contribute to information overload, leading to stress rather than alleviating it. It's essential to choose tools that complement your lifestyle and not dictate it. Technology should enhance the journey, not overshadow the holistic aspects of health and well-being.

In choosing the right tools, personalization is key. Assess your unique needs: are you someone who needs constant feedback to stay motivated, or do you prefer occasional check-ins to ensure you're on track? Aligning your personality and preferences with the capabilities of a tool will lead to better adherence and, ultimately, success. Testing out a few different apps or gadgets on a trial basis can help in making an informed choice.

For those wary of investing in gadgets, many apps offer free versions or trial periods. It allows for experimenting without the pressure of a financial commitment. Often, the foundational features in these free versions are sufficient for someone starting their weight loss journey. Remember, the aim is to build habits that last well beyond the interface of an application.

Ultimately, the right combination of apps and gadgets serves not just as a means to an end but as an empowering toolkit for understanding and optimizing your body. They offer objectivity in a journey that can be emotionally charged, providing a neutral ground for assessing progress. When paired with a supportive community and a balanced mindset, they lay the groundwork for a healthier lifestyle.

As we navigate this nuanced landscape of digital fitness aids, it's clear they are most effective when integrated with a comprehensive approach to health. Use them as guides, checkpoints that illuminate the path rather than sole navigators. Tracking success is not merely about knowing where you stand but recognizing how far you've come, and adjusting course as needed for future journeys. Embrace these technological allies in your quest for transformation, knowing that each step tracked isn't just a measure of advance, but a testament to your commitment to change.

Setting Realistic Goals

When it comes to weight loss, one of the most empowering steps you can take is to set realistic goals. It's not just about knowing where you want to end up; it's also about understanding what's feasible and sustainable along the way. Often, people embark on weight loss journeys with lofty aspirations, only to feel overwhelmed or discouraged when those goals aren't quickly met. By setting realistic goals, you anchor your journey in practicality, promoting both patience and persistence.

The first step in setting realistic goals is to align them with your personal lifestyle and needs. Everybody's journey is unique, woven with distinct circumstances such as personal health conditions, lifestyle habits, and schedules. You might only have 30 minutes a day to dedicate to exercise, or you may face dietary restrictions that require a personalized approach to nutrition. Acknowledging these factors not only steers you away from one-size-fits-all solutions but also paves the way for individualized milestones that are both attainable and meaningful.

It's crucial to break down your weight loss goals into smaller, manageable components. This might mean setting weekly or monthly targets rather than solely focusing on the end goal. For instance, aiming to lose two pounds a week is generally considered safe and achievable. These bite-sized objectives serve as building blocks, keeping you motivated and helping you track your progress without becoming discouraged by the bigger picture. Each small victory boosts your confidence and propels you forward.

Additionally, consider integrating behavioral goals alongside your numerical targets. Rather than concentrating only on the number on the scale, think about the habits you want to change or develop. For instance, you might set a goal to prepare homemade meals five nights a week, reduce your consumption of sugary drinks, or incorporate a new physical activity into your routine. Focusing on such behavioral changes can provide a sense of accomplishment that isn't tied solely to weight, making your journey more fulfilling.

While determination is a powerful tool, flexibility is equally essential. Life is unpredictable, and unexpected challenges—whether they're related to work, health, or family—can disrupt your plans. Instead of viewing these disruptions as setbacks, see them as opportunities to adapt and reaffirm your commitment to your goals. A flexible mindset allows for adjustments without the guilt that often accompanies perceived failures. It's okay to revise your goals to stay aligned with the realities of your life.

An essential part of setting realistic goals is celebrating progress, no matter how small it might seem. Each milestone is a testament to your dedication and is a cause for celebration. Recognition can foster a positive mindset, reinforcing your motivation and commitment. Whether it's fitting into an old pair of jeans or feeling more energetic throughout the day, celebrating these moments can provide the fuel you need to keep going.

Finally, while setting realistic goals is about staying grounded, don't be afraid to dream big. Let your long-term vision be ambitious enough to inspire you, while ensuring your short-term steps are clear and practical. This dual approach maintains your momentum and excitement while keeping you firmly on track toward sustainable results. Surround yourself with reminders of why you embarked on this journey, whether through vision boards, journals, or supportive communities. Let these ignite your passion and remind you of your greater purpose on days when motivation wanes.

Remember, realistic goals are not limitations. They're stepping stones that lead you toward your healthiest, most empowered self. By focusing on what's feasible, celebrating each success, and staying adaptable, you construct a roadmap tailored for long-term success. This journey isn't about deprivation or drastic changes; rather, it's about making purposeful decisions that enrich your life, bolster your well-being, and guide you toward lasting transformation.

How to Create Achievable Milestones Progress can only be meaningful if it's tied to goals that are both ambitious and realistic. In the pursuit of effective weight loss, setting incremental, achievable milestones helps keep focus sharp and motivation high. These milestones serve as tangible checkpoints that align with your overall weight loss goals, ensuring that the journey is comprehensible and less overwhelming. We often underestimate the power of small achievements, yet these are the building blocks of lasting success in any significant life change.

When setting realistic goals for weight loss, it's essential to break these down into smaller, actionable steps. Think of milestones not just as targets, but as mini-celebrations en route to your ultimate goal. Each milestone represents progress and provides the confidence boost necessary to press forward. Begin with a clear understanding of your long-term objective. Whether it's losing a specific amount of weight, fitting into a particular piece of clothing, or simply feeling healthier, that overarching goal gives context to each milestone. The first step in creating achievable milestones is specificity. Vague goals like "lose weight" or "get fit" lack the precision needed to spark action. Instead, aim for clear, measurable objectives. For example, "lose 5 pounds in a month," "run a mile without stopping by December," or "prepare a home-cooked meal five times a week." When goals are specific, progress is easier to track, and the steps needed to achieve them are more apparent. Equally important is ensuring that your milestones are realistic. This means setting targets that are challenging yet attainable within the given timeframe and your lifestyle constraints. Drastic changes can lead to burnout or discouragement. Instead, focus on progress over perfection. Remember, the journey towards weight loss is as much about growth and learning as it is about hitting numbers. Setting achievable milestones that accommodate your current habits and commitments ensures you're moving forward at a manageable pace.

Initially, setting short-term milestones can help build momentum. These are the quick wins that pump up your motivation and lay a strong foundation for long-term habits. Short-term milestones could involve dietary changes, like integrating more vegetables into daily meals or cutting back on sugary drinks. These bite-sized goals are crucial because they furnish rapid feedback, showing that change is possible and probationary efforts are paying off. Once short-term milestones begin to accumulate, it's time to incorporate medium-term goals that bridge the gap to long-term success. These might include goals such as losing a certain percentage of body weight over several months or advancing from walking to jogging regularly. Medium-term milestones gauge progress over an extended period and help test the durability of the changes you're implementing. To keep them effective, continuously reassess these goals against current progress and external circumstances. One vital element in this process is flexibility. Life is unpredictable, and sometimes even the best-laid plans require adjustments. It's important to be adaptable and reassess your milestones if they start to seem unattainable due to unforeseen challenges. Flexibility doesn't equate to lowering all your standards but rather involves a reassessment that ensures your goals remain challenging yet within reach.

Maintaining accountability is crucial for realizing these milestones. Whether through a journal, mobile app, or an accountability partner, tracking both achievements and setbacks helps maintain focus. It also offers a retrospective view that allows for reflection on what strategies worked well and what might need adjustments. Keeping a tangible record of your journey can offer solace during tough phases and add to a sense of accomplishment upon reaching a milestone.

As you set out to create these milestones, visualize each one as a stepping stone in a larger journey. Reflect on why each milestone is important to you personally and how it contributes to the transformative process you're undertaking. This intrinsic connection to your goals keeps motivation from waning and infuses every achievement with deeper meaning. Each milestone reached is not merely a step closer to your goal but a significant part of the change you're making in your lifestyle.

Once a milestone is achieved, celebrate it. Rewarding yourself reinforces the positive behavior and encourages further commitment. It helps create a positive association with goal-setting and completion, making future milestones more exciting rather than burdensome. These celebrations don't have to be extravagant; they can be as simple as a rest day, cooking a favorite meal, or spending time with loved ones.

Finally, remember that this process isn't about a race to the finish line but rather about sustainable, lifelong journey. Long after the goals have been reached, the habits built during this time will continue to influence your health and well-being. Each milestone represents not just a completed task but progress towards a healthier lifestyle, showing that with each step taken thoughtfully, sustainable weight loss is genuinely achievable.

Creating achievable milestones isn't simply about following a step-by-step manual but involves listening to your body and adapting as needed. It's a dynamic process that calls for introspection, discipline, and enthusiasm. By approaching each milestone with intention, patience, and understanding, you fortify the path ahead, enriching both the journey and the destination.

Chapter 10: Overcoming Plateaus

At some point in every weight loss journey, progress seems to stall. These stalls, known as plateaus, are a natural part of the process, but they can be incredibly frustrating. You've been diligent, maintained your routine, yet the scale just won't budge. It can feel like all your efforts are in vain. But take a deep breath — reaching a plateau can be a sign that your body is adjusting to a healthier state. You're not alone in this, and this chapter is here to help guide you through these moments.

Firstly, let's understand what's happening. A plateau occurs when your body's energy balance shifts. Initially, the weight loss journey often reflects rapid changes as water weight decreases and initial fat loss occurs. But as you lose weight, your metabolic rate can slow down because lighter bodies require fewer calories. This natural adaptation can lead to a period where the scale doesn't move, even though you're doing everything right.

So, how do you break through? One strategy is to refresh your exercise routine. Introducing new activities can reignite your metabolism and challenge different muscle groups. Consider adding strength training if you're doing mostly cardio, or vice versa. Changing intensity and duration can also provide the needed stimulus to get past a sticking point. In essence, it might be time to shake things up a bit.

Your dietary habits deserve a closer look too. Sometimes, it's easy to fall into patterns, and perhaps the portion sizes have snuck up or there's mindless snacking that wasn't there before. Keeping a food journal for a week can illuminate patterns and help identify areas for adjustment. Remember, small tweaks can lead to notable changes.

Don't overlook the emotional aspect too. Motivation can naturally waver, especially when instant results aren't visible. This is a great opportunity to reconnect with your deeper reasons for wanting to lose weight. Reflect on the benefits you've already experienced that can't be measured by a scale: higher energy levels, improved mood, better sleep quality, and more. These are victories, too.

Moreover, finding new motivation often comes from setting smaller, achievable goals. These don't necessarily have to be about weight; they can be about fitness milestones or developing new healthy habits. Celebrating these small successes can help keep your spirits high and momentum intact.

Finally, remember that patience and persistence are your allies. This plateau is merely a brief pause in your journey, rather than a full stop. Often, stepping back, reassessing your habits, and introducing some diversity into your routine can reinvigorate progress. Your body has achieved remarkable things already, and it's capable of so much more. You've got this, and you're on the path to lifelong wellness.

Understanding Weight Loss Plateaus

In the journey of weight loss, hitting a plateau is not just common, it's almost an expected milestone. When you first sail through the excitement of shedding pounds, everything seems possible. Yet, so often, progress screeches to a halt. Understanding why these plateaus occur is crucial to navigating and overcoming them, allowing you to continue on the path to sustainable weight loss.

A weight loss plateau happens when your weight remains constant despite consistent dieting and exercise. It's easy to feel like you're doing everything right and still getting nowhere. The body is a complex ecosystem that constantly seeks equilibrium. Over time, as you lose weight, your body's energy requirements decrease, which can slow down or stall your progress. This adaptive mechanism is partly rooted in our biology—it's as if our bodies are programmed to keep us at a stable weight to conserve energy.

Our metabolism plays a pivotal role in reaching a plateau. As you lose weight, your basal metabolic rate (BMR)—the number of calories your body needs at rest—decreases. This means that the caloric deficit you once had is now smaller or nonexistent, slowing your rate of weight loss. But there's more at play; hormonal changes can also influence these plateaus. Hormones like leptin and ghrelin, which regulate hunger and fullness, adapt to weight loss, often driving an increase in hunger, which can make it challenging to maintain a caloric deficit.

Moreover, weight loss doesn't just come from fat reduction; loss of muscle mass can occur as well. Muscle plays a significant role in how many calories your body burns at rest. Therefore, a drop in muscle mass is an unfortunate and often overlooked consequence of weight loss that contributes to plateaus. Engaging in strength training can help counteract this by preserving or even building muscle while still shedding fat.

Psychological factors shouldn't be underestimated either. Mental fatigue can set in over time, making it harder to stick to your healthy habits. Old patterns of stress eating, particularly if under stress or tired, can sneak back in. This isn't a failure but rather an opportunity to reassess and adjust your strategies. Recognizing that weight loss is a dynamic process that involves both body and mind can empower you to find creative solutions.

Breaking through a plateau involves an individualized approach that includes both dietary and lifestyle changes. It might mean shaking up your exercise routine, recalibrating your calorie intake without under-eating, or honing in on metabolism-boosting foods and activities. The objective is to gently nudge your body out of its comfort zone without resorting to extreme measures that could backfire.

Ultimately, understanding and accepting that plateaus are a natural part of the weight loss process can alleviate frustration. They remind us that persistence is essential, and adaptability is key. By embracing patience and maintaining a focus on long-term health, not just the scale, you can transform setbacks into valuable stepping stones toward your desired goals.

Strategies to Break Through Plateaus can transform the disheartening moment of hitting a weight loss plateau into a pivotal turning point on the path to sustainable success. You've been cruising along with your weight loss journey, feeling good about your progress, and then suddenly, the scale refuses to budge. It's frustrating and can feel like a personal failure, though it's anything but. Understanding weight loss plateaus as a natural part of the journey is crucial. Adopting fresh strategies to break through these plateaus not only revives momentum but also renews your commitment to living a healthier life.

First, let's talk about recalibrating your expectations. Plateaus can set off alarms of doubt, but they don't signal the end of progress—they're an opportunity to recalibrate. The body is remarkably adaptive, which can mean it's simply adjusting to your new lower weight. To outsmart this adaptive nature, consider adjusting your calorie intake. When calories in and calories out find equilibrium, weight loss can stagnate. A slight tweak in calorie consumption, either by eating a bit less or working out a bit more, can jolt the body out of its complacency.

Moreover, when dealing with plateaus, variety becomes your best friend. The body adapts to repetitive exercise routines just as it does to calorie patterns. If you've been steadily walking or running, incorporating new activities like cycling or swimming can engage different muscle groups and challenge your metabolism in fresh ways. Similarly, adding strength training can be a game-changer. Muscles are metabolic powerhouses—more muscle mass means more calories burned at rest. Shaking up your routine keeps both your body and mind engaged, preventing the boredom that can accompany repetitive workouts. Think of this plateau phase as an opportunity for profound personal discovery and growth. Ask yourself why you're feeling stuck and how you can leverage this realization. This process involves being honest about your habits and identifying potential blind spots. Perhaps your cheat day has slowly morphed into a cheat weekend, or maybe stress is leading to unacknowledged emotional eating. Embrace this moment, not as a setback but as a learning experience—one in which you learn more about yourself and your needs.

Sometimes what you need isn't more action but deeper rest. Quality sleep is a dynamic player in breaking through plateaus, influencing hormone levels that regulate hunger and metabolism. If you're constantly tired or stressed, the body may hold onto weight despite calorie cuts. Prioritizing sleep can revitalize your mental and physical energy, rebalancing hormones that support weight management. Similarly, stress management cannot be overstated—too much stress and insufficient relaxation dictating your days can lead the body to cling to its reserves.

Additionally, recalibrate your mindset. Recognize that the journey is more than just numbers on a scale; it's about becoming stronger, healthier, more resilient. Embrace progress in other forms—maybe you're lifting more weight at the gym, running a little longer without getting winded, or experiencing more energy throughout the day. Focusing solely on the scale can obscure pivotal non-scale victories critical for maintaining motivation. Cherish these achievements as they too signify substantial personal transformation.

Peer support can't be underestimated. Find someone—whether a friend, a community, or a professional—who can offer guidance and accountability. Sharing your experiences and challenges with others can provide fresh perspectives and rejuvenate motivation. Feedback from a dietitian or personal trainer can offer personalized suggestions that you might not have considered. Open yourself to different viewpoints, and you might discover unexpected solutions to bust through your plateau.

Reassess your macro and micronutrient intake. Sometimes, adjusting the balance of carbohydrates, proteins, and fats can reignite your metabolism. Macronutrients play different roles in energy production and satiety; finding your optimal balance can optimize energy expenditure and satisfy hunger cues more effectively. Likewise, investigating micronutrient intake—ensuring you're not deficient in essential vitamins or minerals—supports the body's ability to function optimally.

Another thrilling aspect is embracing mindfulness practices that connect you more deeply to your body's signals. Mindful eating, for instance, can prevent overeating by encouraging you to listen to your body's hunger and fullness cues. As you become more attuned to these signals, you might find that the small, unconscious habits contributing to plateaus can be recognized and adjusted. Slowing down and savoring each meal shifts focus from external validations—like the scale—to internal contentment and self-awareness.

In the grand scheme of weight loss plateaus, mindset is probably the greatest determinant of success. An optimistic view of this obstacle can shift it from a source of frustration to an invitation for growth. Invite curiosity into your journey; ask yourself what adjustments, however small, could nudge you forward. Each attempt, whether or not immediately successful, teaches you more about what your body and mind need to thrive.

Ultimately, breaking through a plateau requires a mixture of strategy, patience, and self-empathy. It's vital to recognize and celebrate small victories along the way, keeping the focus on long-term health rather than transient setbacks. Stay committed to the belief that with each plateau overcome, you're creating not just a lighter version of yourself, but also a stronger, wiser, and more vibrant one. The path may not always be linear, but with the right strategies and a resilient mindset, you will move forward.

Staying Motivated During Setbacks

Plateaus in weight loss can feel like standing on a treadmill going nowhere fast. You've put in the effort, and yet, the results seem to stall. So, how do you keep the momentum going when the scale refuses to budge? It's crucial to remember that setbacks aren't failures; they're the body's way of adapting to change. This is your body's natural response to the progress you've already made, and it's an opportunity to recalibrate and push forward with renewed determination.

Motivation can wane when faced with setbacks, but shifting your mindset can make all the difference. Instead of viewing a plateau as a roadblock, see it as a detour. This is a chance to explore new routes on your journey to weight loss. Maybe it's time to revisit your eating habits or switch up your exercise routine. Keeping things fresh not only challenges your body but keeps your mind engaged and motivated. Variety can be the spice that reawakens your enthusiasm and propels you past this temporary halt.

It's also important to reiterate the power of small victories. When progress seems to halt, take a moment to recognize what you've already achieved. Celebrate the healthful habits you've incorporated into your life or the stamina you've built. Sometimes, these victories are more significant than a number on a scale. Keeping a journal or a simple list of these milestones can remind you of how far you've come and how capable you are of going even further.

Engaging with a supportive community can also reignite your motivation. Sharing your journey with friends or groups who understand the challenge can provide emotional support and practical advice. They can offer encouragement when you need it most and help you brainstorm new strategies to break through the plateau. There's magic in having cheerleaders by your side who believe in your potential even when you doubt it yourself.

Remember, intrinsic motivation born from personal values and internal desires tends to be more sustainable than external rewards. Reflect on why you started this journey in the first place. Did you want increased energy, better health, or to feel more comfortable in your own skin? Reconnecting with your deeper motivations can reignite the passion needed to push through difficult times.

Occasionally, setbacks necessitate a bit of patience and self-compassion. It's easy to be harsh on yourself when things don't go as planned, but developing a kind internal dialogue can be empowering. Treating yourself with kindness means acknowledging that plateaus are a natural part of any growth process, not an indication of your worth or effort. This self-compassion will not only enhance your motivation but also make your journey more enjoyable.

Finally, visualize success—not just the end goal but the entire experience. Visualize feeling stronger, more confident, and healthier. Daydream about climbing that hill or running that extra mile effortlessly. This mental exercise can foster resilience and give you the emotional boost needed to keep going. By nurturing a positive mental image, you cultivate the inner strength to overcome setbacks and continue towards your weight loss goals.

Maintaining Focus and Determination in the journey of weight loss is often likened to navigating a long and winding road. This path, at times strewn with obstacles and unexpected turns, demands a steadfast focus and an unwavering determination. Overcoming plateaus, especially when facing setbacks, requires more than just a change in tactics; it involves cultivating a mindset resilient to the trials that inevitably arise. By setting realistic and manageable goals, we can keep our eyes on the horizon without letting temporary setbacks derail our progress.

Setbacks aren't just bumps in the road—they're opportunities to learn and grow. Each challenge presents a chance to reassess and recalibrate. When you hit a plateau, it's easy to feel discouraged, yet maintaining focus at this juncture is crucial. It's vital to remind yourself why you embarked on this journey in the first place. Refresh your commitment by reflecting on your motivations and the benefits that await you beyond the plateau. Think of it as a reset button, not a dead end.

Emotional resilience plays a key role in sustaining determination. Life doesn't conveniently pause for us when we're on a weight loss journey. Stressful events and changes in routine can easily sap your motivation. To counteract this, develop a toolkit for emotional well-being. Incorporate practices like journaling, meditative breathing, or short daily walks to calm the mind. These small habits anchor your day and provide clarity, helping maintain focus even amidst chaos.

Creating a routine that supports your goals can also help in maintaining focus. Consistency is often the antidote to wavering determination. Design a daily schedule that aligns with your weight loss objectives, whether it's meal prepping on Sundays or setting aside time for a morning workout. By establishing a predictable rhythm, you create a supportive environment that's conducive to success. Remember, it's the repeated actions over time that lead to the most profound changes.

Sometimes, maintaining focus means narrowing it. We often spread ourselves thin, juggling multiple changes at once. This can dilute our efforts and lead to burnout. Instead, prioritize one key behavior change at a time. Perhaps it's as simple as increasing your daily water intake or dedicating an extra 10 minutes to physical activity. By concentrating your efforts, you bolster your determination, making it more likely to achieve and sustain your goals.

Community can be a powerful motivator when you hit a plateau. Isolation can breed discouragement, so seek support from those who understand your journey. This might involve joining a local fitness class or finding an online community where you can share experiences and strategies. The encouragement and accountability from others can ignite your resolve and help you maintain focus. You're not in this alone; others are on this path with you, cheering you on.

In addition, celebrate small victories. Every step forward, no matter how minor it seems, deserves recognition. These moments reinforce your focus and invigorate your resolve. Whether it's fitting into an old pair of jeans or opting for a healthier snack, take a moment to honor your progress. These celebrations keep you grounded in positivity and remind you of your capabilities.

An often overlooked aspect of maintaining focus is the role of self-compassion. Be gentle with yourself, especially during setbacks. Berating yourself for not meeting your ideals only saps energy and determination. Instead, approach setbacks with curiosity rather than judgment. Ask yourself what can be learned from the experience and how you can apply these lessons moving forward. This mindset not only keeps you focused but also fosters personal growth.

Furthermore, visualizing success can serve as a powerful tool. Spend a few moments each day imagining yourself achieving your weight loss goals. Visualize the energy, confidence, and health you desire. This mental imagery can reinforce your focus, serving as a reminder of why maintaining determination is crucial. It keeps your goals tangible and within reach.

Finally, embrace flexibility in your approach. Maintaining focus doesn't mean rigid adherence to one path; rather, it's about perseverance with adaptability. Life's unpredictability means that sometimes plans need to change. Be open to adjusting strategies when necessary, whether that means trying a new workout, experimenting with meal plans, or recalibrating expectations. This adaptability not only keeps you focused but also resilient in the face of setbacks.

In sum, staying motivated and determined throughout setbacks and plateaus involves a multifaceted approach. It's about nurturing your mental health, creating supportive routines, and building a network of encouragement. By embracing these strategies, you reinforce your commitment and ensure that your focus remains steadfast—even when the road gets tough. With determination, every challenge becomes an opportunity to step further into the life you've envisioned for yourself.

Chapter 11: Long-term Lifestyle Changes

Embracing long-term lifestyle changes might feel like a daunting endeavor, but it's the secret sauce to achieving sustainable weight loss. A shift in mindset is crucial here. We're not talking about transient fixes or temporary diet plans that evaporate with the first signs of success. Instead, it's about cultivating new habits that blend seamlessly into everyday life, almost like they were meant to be there all along.

The cornerstone of this transformation lies in establishing sustainable eating habits. This doesn't mean rigid dieting but rather creating a balanced diet plan that suits your unique needs and preferences. Begin by incorporating a range of whole foods, rich in nutrients, that fuel your body efficiently without depriving you of culinary joy. Consistency, not perfection, is key. It's about making small, incremental changes so they become second nature over time.

Imagine the power of integrating regular physical activity into your routine. It doesn't have to be strenuous or time-consuming; what's important is the consistency. Choose activities that you enjoy—be it walking, dancing, swimming, or cycling—turning exercise from a chore into an extension of your day. The goal is to make movement a habit that doesn't require a second thought.

Life's unpredictability means that flexibility is a crucial part of this journey. You'll encounter holidays, celebrations, and stress. There will be times when you stray from these new routines, and that's perfectly okay. The measure of success is not in never faltering, but in how quickly you return to your path after a detour. Maintain a compassionate perspective towards yourself, ensuring your inner dialogue echoes kindness and understanding.

Support systems play a pivotal role in this transformation. Whether it's family, friends, or a community of like-minded individuals, having a network that encourages and inspires can boost your resolve. They provide a safety net, and their encouragement can reinvigorate your spirits when motivation wanes.

This chapter isn't about dictating what you should eat or prescribing specific workouts. Rather, it illuminates a path for crafting a lifestyle that doesn't feel restrictive but liberating. It's about tuning in to your body's needs, understanding your triggers, and navigating obstacles with resilience. You're not alone on this journey, and the road doesn't have to be perfect—just persistent.

Ultimately, long-term lifestyle change is a personal evolution. With each mindful choice, each step forward, you're building a life aligned with your values and aspirations. It's a celebration of progress, however small, amassing over time into profound transformation. And with every victory, you're not just succeeding in weight loss; you're thriving in a life that reflects who you truly are and what you desire to become.

Establishing Sustainable Eating Habits

In our pursuit of lasting weight loss, establishing sustainable eating habits is crucial. It's about making choices that nourish both the body and mind, leading to a healthier, happier life. Sustainable eating isn't about adhering to rigid diet plans or depriving yourself of the foods you enjoy. Instead, it's about creating a balanced approach that fits into your daily life and supports your long-term goals. To make these changes stick, it's essential to focus on consistency rather than perfection.

The key to sustainable eating is understanding what your body truly needs. This involves recognizing hunger cues and distinguishing them from cravings or emotional urges. It's about learning to listen to your body and feeding it with nutrient-rich foods that fuel your energy and keep you satisfied. This means embracing a variety of food groups, including fruits, vegetables, whole grains, lean proteins, and healthy fats. Creating a well-rounded plate not only supports weight loss but also promotes overall health.

Mindful eating plays a significant role in establishing these habits. By paying attention to what and how much you eat, you develop a greater appreciation for your meals and can better sense when you're full. Mindful eating involves slowing down, chewing thoroughly, and savoring each bite. It helps break the cycle of mindless snacking and promotes a deeper connection with your food. When you focus less on restrictions and more on enjoyment and nourishment, eating becomes a more pleasurable and sustainable experience.

Planning and preparation are also important components of sustainable eating. Taking the time to plan your meals for the week can prevent impulsive eating and reduce the temptation to opt for convenience foods. Exploring new recipes or meal prepping can simplify your routine and ensure you have healthy choices readily available. This approach not only helps guide better food choices but also saves time and stress in the long run.

Incorporating flexibility into your eating habits is equally vital. Life is unpredictable, and strict rules can lead to frustration and setbacks. Allow yourself the freedom to adapt when necessary, whether it's attending social gatherings or handling unexpected events. By being flexible, you can enjoy these moments without feeling guilty or derailing your progress. It's all about balance and finding what works for you, even when life throws curveballs.

Ultimately, establishing sustainable eating habits involves a shift in mindset. It's about cultivating a positive relationship with food and viewing it as a tool for well-being, rather than a source of stress or restriction. This mindset empowers you to make choices that align with your values and goals, fostering a healthier lifestyle that is both attainable and enjoyable. By focusing on the journey rather than the end result, you're more likely to achieve lasting success in your weight loss efforts.

Creating a Balanced Diet Plan is about much more than counting calories or following the latest food trend. It's a cornerstone of establishing sustainable eating habits, focusing on nourishment and variety rather than restriction. This isn't just about losing weight; it's about creating a holistic life change that enhances well-being and promotes long-lasting health. A balanced diet plan can help eliminate the anxiety often associated with eating by providing structure and clarity. It becomes a self-empowered choice, a series of informed decisions that offer freedom rather than limitation. Let's explore how to construct this crucial aspect of a long-term lifestyle change.

At the heart of a balanced diet plan is the idea of moderation and variety. This means including all food groups in your meals: proteins, carbohydrates, fats, fruits, vegetables, and even the occasional treat. When you embrace the diversity in nature's bounty, you not only satisfy your taste buds but also ensure that your body receives a wide range of nutrients essential for optimal health. This buffet of nutrients supports metabolic processes, aids in repairing tissues, and powers your day-to-day activities. Moreover, once you remove the stigma of "bad" foods, the guilt associated with eating can diminish. You're left with a more joyful dining experience and a healthier relationship with food.

One effective strategy is to think of your diet as a pie chart, not too dissimilar from those we've all seen in nutritional guides. Ideally, half of this chart is devoted to vegetables and fruits, grown abundantly and harvested at their peak for flavor and nutrition. A quarter is reserved for whole grains such as brown rice, quinoa, or oats. While the remaining quarter is a source of protein, think variety here—lean meats, fish, beans, or plant-based options each bring something valuable to the table, literally and metaphorically.

Transitioning to this balanced approach doesn't happen overnight. It involves gradually shifting away from processed foods, which often lure us in with convenience and addictive flavors, and moving towards more whole-food options. This transformation isn't about precision but progress. Small, gradual adjustments provide room to adapt, preventing the feeling of being overwhelmed that often accompanies drastic dietary changes. These incremental shifts also pave the way for habit-building, a cornerstone for any lifestyle change meant to last.

A balanced plate is not a static concept—seasonal variations play a significant role. Our bodies often crave different foods at different times of the year. Summer might spark a desire for fresh salads and grilled vegetables, while fall might invite heartier meals such as roasted root vegetables and warming spices. Listening to these natural inclinations can enhance the satisfaction of eating, ensuring that meals are never monotonous.

Fluid balance should be part of the diet plan, though it often doesn't receive the attention it deserves. Adequate hydration supports every cellular process in the body, aiding digestion, nutrient transport, and even the regulation of appetite. Aiming to drink water or herbal teas throughout the day can prevent the common mistake of translating thirst cues into hunger pangs, reducing unnecessary calorie intake.

Cravings will happen; they're a natural part of being human. The key is to manage them mindfully without giving in impulsively. Recognize them as signals from your body, often requests for a nutrient that might be in deficit. For example, a chocolate craving might indicate a need for magnesium. Instead of shunning these cravings, honor them by allowing occasional indulgences in moderate portions—these could be moments for mindful eating, where fully engaging with your senses in the eating experience allows for satisfaction without overconsumption.

Meal planning can play an instrumental role in sticking to a balanced diet plan. Taking a bit of time each week to map out meals can reduce stress and save time, providing a roadmap for nutritious and balanced eating. It's like setting an intention for the week ahead and increases the likelihood of resisting last-minute unhealthy choices. The shopping list derived from a meal plan ensures you stock your kitchen with only the essentials and keeps you on track financially too.

Ultimately, a balanced diet doesn't have to be an intricate puzzle. It's about listening to your body, aligning with nature, and allowing yourself the grace to enjoy food. As you lay down this foundation, you'll discover not just physical transformation but a shift in mindset. Words like "diet" take on a new meaning, one that is not synonymous with sacrifice but instead reflects choice, nourishment, and empowerment.

Integrating Regular Physical Activity

Incorporating regular physical activity into your lifestyle isn't just a recommendation—it's a transformative choice that can redefine your approach to health and wellness. Exercise is more than just a tool for weight management; it's a way to energize your body and mind. The journey towards integrating physical activity into your everyday routine starts with a shift in mindset. It's about embracing movement as a vital part of life rather than a chore you need to check off your list.

Start by finding activities you genuinely enjoy. Whether it's dancing, hiking, swimming, or joining a local yoga class, the key is to choose something that makes you feel good. When you engage in activities that you love, you're more likely to stick with them in the long run. Think of physical activity as a celebration of what your body can do, and not just a way to burn calories. This perspective not only lightens the emotional weight around exercise but also encourages consistency.

Integrating regular movement can be as simple as making small changes to your daily routine. Consider opting for the stairs over the elevator, or a brisk walk during lunch breaks. These incremental changes add up and can significantly enhance your physical stamina. As you steadily increase your activity level, try not to focus solely on the physical benefits. Instead, pay attention to how movement affects your mood and energy levels. Physical activity releases endorphins, which play a crucial role in improving mental health and well-being.

Community engagement can also be a powerful motivator when integrating regular physical exercise. Joining a group, whether it's a cycling club or a running group, can provide a sense of camaraderie and accountability. Exercising with others can encourage you through moments of doubt and push you further than you'd go alone. The shared goals and collective achievements can transform what might feel like a task into an enjoyable and consistent ritual.

In the process of incorporating exercise, it's vital to pay attention to your body's signals. Days of rest are as important as days of movement. Listen to your body and its needs to avoid burnout or injury. Rest does not equate to inactivity but rather is an integral part of building a sustainable physical routine. Alternating days of high-intensity workouts with lighter activities like stretching or leisurely walks can provide balance and prevent exhaustion.

Remember, the goal is sustainable integration of physical activity into your lifestyle, not short-lived bursts of intense exercise. It's all about creating habits that fit smoothly into your life without overwhelming it. With patience and perseverance, regular physical activity can become a gratifying and indispensable component of your life. As you progress, you'll likely notice not just changes in your physical health, but also a keener sense of empowerment that extends beyond the limits of a daily workout.

Making Exercise a Daily Habit Integrating regular physical activity into your life isn't just about fitness; it's about embracing a shift towards a healthier, more energetic you. The journey of transforming exercise into a daily habit can be as rewarding as it is challenging. Understanding how to make this transition smoothly is crucial to achieving long-term lifestyle changes. It requires patience, persistence, and a bit of strategy to naturally weave physical activity into the fabric of your daily routine.

Consider this: our bodies are designed to move, and when we integrate physical activity into our daily lives, it nourishes our bodies and minds. The goal isn't to run marathons or spend countless hours in the gym. Instead, it's about finding what works for you, what fits seamlessly into your life, and what you'll enjoy enough to keep doing, day in and day out. The key to making exercise a habit lies in understanding and aligning it with your personal values and lifestyle.

Starting small can make a significant impact. Think of exercise as a series of small, manageable steps rather than a daunting task. Begin with simple activities that you can easily incorporate into your day. This might be a brisk walk during lunch breaks, a short yoga session in the morning, or a dance class with friends in the evening. As these small actions become part of your routine, they'll stop feeling like 'exercise' and start feeling like a natural, pleasurable part of your day.

Setting clear, achievable goals can also play a pivotal role in developing a daily exercise routine. When you map out what you want to achieve with your physical activity, it gives you a purpose to stay committed. These goals should be specific, measurable, and tailored to your personal aspirations. Whether it's walking a certain number of steps daily or spending a certain amount of time being active, having a goal gives you something to strive for, making the habit-forming process more tangible and rewarding.

On days when motivation wanes, remind yourself why you started. Link your exercise routine to something deeply personal—perhaps it's the joy of feeling more energetic, the confidence in achieving a healthier weight, or the aspiration to set a positive example for your family. These deeper motivations can serve as powerful reminders of why integrating daily exercise is important and help reignite your commitment when the going gets tough.

Another effective strategy is to incorporate variety to prevent monotony and burnout. Keep things interesting by trying different activities that excite you. Cycling today, hiking tomorrow, swimming the next day—you get the idea. Exploring different forms of movement not only keeps your routine fresh and exciting but also helps your body become more adaptable and resilient. This adaptability can improve all-around fitness, making exercise even more enjoyable as you recognize the benefits it brings.

Community and accountability can further enhance your efforts toward making exercise a daily habit. Engage with friends, family, or local groups that share your interest in being active. Finding a workout buddy not only makes the experience more enjoyable but also adds a layer of responsibility. You'll be less likely to skip a workout if you know someone else is counting on you to show up. Plus, sharing your achievements and challenges can strengthen your connections with others striving for similar goals.

Technology can be an ally in these efforts, offering apps and wearable devices that track your activity levels, set reminders, and celebrate your milestones. These tools provide valuable insights into your progress and help you visualize your growth over time. They can also help make fitness feel more personalized and integrated into your daily life without being intrusive or overwhelming.

As you integrate regular physical activity into your life, remember that consistency trumps intensity. It's more beneficial to engage in moderate activity daily than to engage in intense sessions sparingly. This consistent engagement helps seal the habit, gradually transforming it into a non-negotiable part of your lifestyle. When exercise is consistent, and feels as normal as brushing your teeth or drinking your morning coffee, you've succeeded in making it a lasting habit.

Reflect on your journey frequently and be kind to yourself. Acknowledge how far you've come, celebrate every small win, and don't be too hard on yourself if you miss a day. Life is unpredictable and some days won't go as planned, but a missed workout is only a setback if it derails your long-term commitment. Use these reflections as opportunities to adjust your approach, drawing closer to discovering what truly works for you.

Lastly, keep the bigger picture in focus. You're not just training for today or tomorrow but investing in your long-term health and happiness. Physical activity enhances your quality of life, increasing longevity, reducing the risk of chronic diseases, and improving mental well-being. This investment in yourself is the ultimate goal of making exercise a daily habit—turning short-term actions into lasting health benefits.

By cultivating a routine of daily movement, you're engaging in a powerful form of self-care that nurtures the body and enriches the mind. As you continue on this path, you'll find that exercise is not a burden on your time but a blessing that complements and enhances your life. The journey of making exercise a daily habit is personal and dynamic, interwoven with challenges and triumphs, but ultimately, it's about creating a life where movement is a celebration and a refuge within.

Chapter 12: Inspiring Stories of Transformation

Stories of transformation have a unique power to ignite change in our own lives. They show us what's possible when commitment meets resilience. One such story is about Emily, a young woman who struggled with weight gain for years. It wasn't just about the numbers on the scale for her; it was about regaining control over her life and health. Emily's journey began when she committed to making small, manageable changes. She started by choosing whole foods over processed ones, slowly incorporating regular walks into her daily routine. It wasn't easy at first, but her perseverance paid off. Today, Emily not only looks different but feels renewed and empowered.

Another inspiring account is that of James, who had battled with emotional eating after a traumatic event. Understanding the psychological aspects of his eating habits was a pivotal moment for him. With the support of a therapist, James learned to recognize his triggers and developed healthier coping mechanisms. This story is a testament to the power of mental health support in physical transformation. James didn't just lose weight; he gained a new perspective on life and the strength to face challenges head-on.

Let's not forget Carla, whose transformation came not from weight loss per se, but from embracing a healthier lifestyle. Frustrated by yo-yo dieting and its toll on her body, Carla decided to take a different path. She focused on establishing a balanced approach to nutrition, integrating enjoyable physical activities, and prioritizing self-care. Over time, Carla discovered the joy of living healthily for herself, not for societal expectations. Her story shows us that transformation is deeply personal and goes beyond aesthetics.

These stories serve as poignant reminders that while the journey to weight loss and wellness can be daunting, it's also filled with potential for profound personal growth. Whether it's through gentle habits or the bravery to seek help, each step forward is a victory in itself. Embrace these narratives as catalysts for your own change, because if they can do it, so can you.

Real-life Successes

In the quest for sustainable weight loss, stories of real people overcoming obstacles stand as a beacon of hope and inspiration. These are individuals who, like many, grappled with the complexities of weight loss but found a path that worked for them. Their stories highlight not just the scales tipping in their favor, but the profound personal transformations that accompanied shedding those pounds.

One such success story is of Samantha, a mother of two who found herself overwhelmed by stress and time constraints. Balancing her job and family seemed impossible, let alone squeezing in time for herself. By committing to gradual changes, like taking daily walks and choosing home-cooked meals over takeout, she not only lost weight but also regained her energy and confidence. Samantha's journey reminds us that the most impactful changes are often rooted in simplicity and consistency.

Then there's Carlos, who had tried every fad diet under the sun, only to end up in an endless cycle of weight fluctuations. It wasn't until he approached weight loss with a mindset of understanding his eating habits and emotions that things changed. By incorporating mindful eating practices and building a supportive network of friends and family, Carlos achieved a transformation that was both physical and emotional. His story emphasizes the importance of tackling the psychological aspects of eating and surrounding oneself with encouragement and support.

Finally, consider the triumphant journey of James, a retired veteran who battled with weight gain after leaving the service. He found that a combination of strength training and community engagement became his pillars of success. By setting small, realistic goals and celebrating each victory, James exemplified how perseverance and a shift in lifestyle can lead to lasting results. His experience serves as a testimony that true transformation isn't just about the body—it's about redefining one's life.

Learning from Others' Journeys offers an intimate look into the lives of those who have walked the path you're considering—or are currently navigating. When you take a moment to examine the journeys of others, you gain insights that textbooks and theories can't always provide. This section is about finding a sense of community in the diverse experiences of real individuals who have achieved sustainable weight loss. Their stories serve as a touchstone for those who seek change, a reminder that the battles fought are not just theirs alone, but shared by many.

Imagine, for a moment, a woman named Sarah who's faced numerous hurdles on her weight loss journey. Her story isn't about a sudden, exhilarating transformation but rather a gradual, steady metamorphosis that's been as much about mental resilience as it has been about physical health. She began with small steps, rejecting crash diets and instead, opting for balanced nutrition combined with moderate exercise. The significant shift for Sarah came from her realization that weight loss wasn't a temporary project but an enduring lifestyle change. Her journey reminds us that perseverance, not perfection, is key in the quest for health.

Similarly, there's Mark, whose path to weight loss was paved with social support and accountability. With the encouragement of friends and family, he embraced a routine of activities that fulfilled him—be it a walk in the park or a hike in the mountains. Mark's experience highlights the impact of a robust support network in making lifestyle changes stick. It's an empowering reminder that while the journey is personal, the backing of those who believe in your potential makes a profound difference.

Learning from others' journeys doesn't just show you what works—it reveals the setbacks and failures along the way. Consider Emma, who initially saw weight loss as a series of strict dietary restrictions. Her transformation stalled under the pressure of these limits, leading her back to square one multiple times. It was only when she learned to listen to her body's signals and accepted an adaptive, rather than punitive, approach that she began to see sustainable progress. Emma's experiences underline the importance of self-compassion and understanding in overcoming perceived failures.

It's vital to recognize that each person's journey is distinctly their own, shaped by unique circumstances, challenges, and discoveries. Yet, the essence of their stories carries universal truths that can be adapted to fit any individual's context. When you hear about James, who found solace in mindful eating and meditation, you realize that the methods employed can be as varied as the people themselves. What matters is finding what resonates with you, adapting lessons from others to nourish your body and mind concurrently.

The power in learning from others lies not in imitation, but in adaptation and personalization. No two journeys are identical, and what succeeds for one might not for another. However, the mosaic of experiences forms a compelling picture that collectively conveys the message: sustainable change is possible. These stories provide a framework, one where success is built on realistic goals, consistent actions, and an unwavering commitment to self-betterment.

In a world filled with overwhelming diet trends and fitness fads, the practical wisdom gleaned from real-life successes acts as both a beacon and a balm. It's about finding inspiration and realizing that, although the road ahead may be daunting, you are not traveling it alone. Others have forged ahead—they've stumbled, and risen again. Through their triumphs and tribulations, they remind us that the destination is not just about shedding pounds, but about gaining a healthier, happier life.

Your journey toward weight loss is as unique as your fingerprint, yet intrinsically linked to the shared human experience. As you learn from others, you draw strength from their triumphs and courage from their challenges. Embrace these stories not as step-by-step guides but as narratives of empowerment. In reflecting on others' journeys, you may well find the key to unlocking your own path to transformation. Take these lessons to heart, and let them fuel your own inspiring story of change.

Conclusion

As we reach the conclusion of our exploration into effective and sustainable weight loss, it's important to pause and reflect on the transformative journey you've embarked upon. Weight loss, as we've uncovered, isn't just about shedding pounds; it's a profound change in how we live, think, and engage with the world each day. Standing on this new horizon, let's take a moment to appreciate how far we've come and gaze ahead at the endless possibilities that lie before us.

In this journey, you've equipped yourself with a wealth of knowledge. Understanding the science of metabolism has allowed you to tune into your body's unique rhythms. You've learned about the vital role genetics play while recognizing the immense power of lifestyle choices. And, perhaps most importantly, you're now aware that there is no one-size-fits-all solution. Embracing individuality and understanding your own body is key to achieving lasting results.

The nutritional truths you've discovered have shown that balance is not just a dietary preference, but a foundational pillar of health. You've seen past the allure of quick-fix fad diets and embraced the virtues of real, whole foods. Through nourishment, you're fostering a relationship with food that respects both your needs and wants, leading you toward sustainable change.

Exercise has emerged not merely as a means to an end but as a joyful expression of what your body is capable of achieving. From optimized cardio routines to the power of strength training, active living contributes to your overall sense of well-being, boosting not only your metabolism but your mood and outlook on life as well.

We've delved into the intricate link between mind and body, exploring the psychology of eating and the impact of emotional triggers. With this awareness, you're cultivating mindful eating habits that align with your goals, transforming how you interact with food and how you nurture yourself in both good times and bad.

Alongside healthy eating and movement, the essential roles of sleep and stress management have been elevated within your understanding of health. Recognizing how profoundly these elements impact weight and wellness ensures you support your body holistically, promoting harmony between rest, stress resilience, and daily activity.

We've also shed light on the invaluable support networks around you—friends, family, and professionals who cheer you on and hold you accountable. Acknowledging that no one has to do this alone empowers you to lean on others when needed, creating a community grounded in empathy and shared triumphs.

Tracking progress and setting realistic goals are not just ways to measure success; they're strategies that encourage continued motivation and resilience. Embracing setbacks as growth opportunities rather than failures allows you to maintain focus, adapting your course while celebrating each incremental achievement.

As life moves forward, you've recognized the necessity of embedding these habits into your daily routines, crafting a lifestyle that feels authentic and sustainable. You know that maintaining change requires intentional practice and the courage to align your actions with your core values daily. Here, transformation becomes a journey of continuous growth.

Drawing inspiration from transformative stories of others who've walked a similar path, you're never short of motivation. These narratives remind you of the power of perseverance, demonstrating that significant changes are not just possible—they're achievable with commitment and heart.

In closing, take pride in this journey. The knowledge gained, and the resilience built are timeless empowering tools. You're stepping into a life sculpted by your own hands, one that resonates with your vision of health and happiness. This isn't a fleeting transformation; it's the unfolding of a more vibrant, mindful, and empowered you. Hold onto this vision as you continue to embrace, discover, and shape the life you desire. Congratulations on reaching this point, not as a conclusion but as the beginning of a lifelong adventure of wellness and self-discovery. Remember, your journey is unique, filled with its own victories and lessons. And as you move forward, continue to be gentle with yourself, celebrating the progress you've made and the aspirations you have yet to fulfill. Here's to your ongoing journey of living well.

Appendix A: Resources and Tools for Weight Loss Success

Embarking on a weight loss journey is more sustainable and effective when you're armed with the right resources and tools. This appendix offers a selection of practical tools and supportive resources designed to help you navigate the path to lasting weight loss success. Harness these assets to empower yourself and stay motivated throughout your journey.

Digital Tools and Apps

In our technology-driven world, digital tools can be game-changers in reaching weight loss goals. Consider incorporating these tools to streamline and enhance your efforts:

- **Calorie and Activity Trackers:** Apps like MyFitnessPal and Lose It! allow you to log meals and exercise, providing insights into caloric intake and expenditures. These apps help you stay accountable and informed.
- **Customizable Workout Plans:** Apple's Fitness+ and other subscription-based platforms offer tailored workout programs. They cater to various fitness levels, ensuring you challenge yourself appropriately.
- **Meditation and Mindfulness Apps:** Headspace and Calm can aid in stress reduction, a critical component of weight loss. They guide you through relaxation techniques and mindful practices, helping you cultivate a healthier relationship with food.

Nutritional Guides and Recipe Resources

Nutrition plays a pivotal role in weight management. Knowing what to eat is as crucial as knowing what to avoid. Arm yourself with these resources:

- **Culinary Blogs:** Sites like Minimalist Baker and EatingWell offer nutritious and delicious recipes that make healthy eating enjoyable and varied.
- **Nutrition Education Websites:** The USDA's MyPlate plan provides guidelines to create balanced meals tailored to individual dietary needs and restrictions.

Community and Support Networks

Having a support system greatly impacts motivation and accountability. Seek out these communities for inspiration and guidance:

- **Online Forums:** Platforms like Reddit's Health and Fitness community offer a space to share experiences, ask questions, and gain insights from others on similar journeys.
- **Social Media Groups:** Joining Facebook groups focused on weight loss can provide support and encouragement, connecting you with people sharing similar aspirations.

Professional Guidance

Nothing substitutes personalized advice from professionals. These resources can connect you with experts to keep you on track:

- **Virtual Consultations:** Services like Teladoc offer direct access to nutritionists and fitness coaches for personalized advice without geographical limitations.

- **Certified Trainers and Nutritionists:** Look for professionals associated with recognized organizations such as the American Council on Exercise (ACE) and the Academy of Nutrition and Dietetics for validated expertise.

Books and Self-help Resources

Navigating the complex world of weight loss is easier with knowledge. Consider these readings to empower and educate yourself:

- **Informative Reads:** Books like Michael Pollan's "In Defense of Food" provide insights into healthy eating habits, dismantling common dietary myths.
- **Motivational Literature:** Works by James Clear, such as "Atomic Habits," offer strategies for developing sustainable habits that support weight loss goals.

Each of these tools and resources can assist you in moving toward a healthier and more fulfilling lifestyle. With commitment and the right support, you can make informed, empowered choices, breaking free from the cycle of fad diets and temporary fixes. Transforming your life one step at a time is not just achievable, it's within your grasp.

9 798345 990735